Tutorials in Clinical Surgery in General
Volume 1

D1809100

To Albert with [illegible] of all regards [handwritten dedication]

Other books by F. G. Smiddy

Tutorial in Surgery 1
F. G. Smiddy

Tutorials in Surgery 2
F. G. Smiddy

Multiple Choice Questions in General Pathology
F. G. Smiddy/J. L. Turk

Pocket Examiner in Pathology
P. N. Cowen/F. G. Smiddy

For Churchill Livingstone:
Publisher: Peter Richardson
Editorial Co-ordination: Editorial Resources Unit
 Copy Editor: Joanna Smith
Production Controller: Neil Dickson
Design: Design Resources Unit
Sales Promotion Executive: Louise Johnstone

Tutorials in Clinical Surgery in General
Volume 1

F. G. Smiddy MD CHM FRCS
Formerly Consultant Surgeon, The General Infirmary Leeds and
Clayton Hospital, Wakefield, UK
Member of the Court of Examiners of the Royal College of Surgeons, England,
Examiner in Pathology

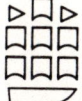
CHURCHILL LIVINGSTONE
EDINBURGH LONDON MELBOURNE NEW YORK AND TOKYO 1991

CHURCHILL LIVINGSTONE
Medical Division of Longman Group UK Limited

Distributed in the United States of America by Churchill
Livingstone Inc., 650 Avenue of the Americas, New York,
N.Y. 10011, and by associated companies, branches and
representatives throughout the world.

© F. G. Smiddy 1991

All rights reserved. No part of this publication may be
reproduced, stored in a retrieval system, or transmitted in any
form or by any means, electronic, mechanical, photocopying,
recording or otherwise, without either the prior permission of
the publishers (Churchill Livingstone, Robert Stevenson
House, 1–3 Baxter's Place, Leith Walk, Edinburgh EH1
3 AF), or a licence permitting restricted copying in the United
Kingdom issued by the Copyright Licensing Agency Ltd,
90 Tottenham Court Road, London, WIP 9HE.

First published 1991

ISBN 0-443-04577-1

British Library Cataloguing in Publication Data
CIP catalogue record for this book is available from the
British Library.

Library of Congress Cataloging in Publication Data
Smiddy, F. G. (Francis Geoffrey)
    Tutorials in clinical surgery in general/F.G. Smiddy.
        p.   cm.
    Includes index.
    ISBN 0-443-04577-1
    1. Surgery, Operative.   I. Title.
    [DNLM: 1. Surgery, Operative.   WU 500 S639t]
RD32.S637   1991
617'.91—dc20
DNLM/DLC
for Library of Congress   91-19392
                                                                         CIP

Printed and bound in Great Britain by
Butler & Tanner Ltd, Frome and London

Preface

The recent reorientation of the Fellowship Examination, with its emphasis on basic principles rather than the minutiae of surgical technique, suggested to the author that a new revision text was required by the candidates. This book is not to be regarded as a textbook of surgery – which it is not in the author's competence to write – but as a series of short notes written on and around the subjects presented in the Guide to the Fellowship recently published by the Royal College of England which brings the subject matter of the examination more into line with that required by the other Colleges.

It is not intended to be comprehensive, but the writer hopes that the reader will find that the great majority of the clinical topics listed in the syllabus are included within this volume.

In due course, it is hoped that a second volume will appear which will cover those topics which are not included in this book.

Leeds, 1991   F.G.S.

To Rebecca and Huw Morgan

Contents

1 Antisepsis and asepsis

HISTORICAL INTRODUCTION

For centuries, the idea that tiny creatures could produce disease had been discussed. Even in the first century B.C., Vano had held the view that certain minute animals, invisible to the naked eye, bred in swampy land and then, borne by the air, reached the inside of the body by way of the mouth and caused disease. In 1530, Girolamo Frascatoro, famed for his poem on syphilis, attributed the spread of the disease to 'seeds of contagion' and even surmised the mode of transmission. In the seventeenth century, Antoni von Leeuwenhoek working with an early microscope described the minute animaculae only to be largely ignored; and by 1795, Alexander Gordon of Aberdeen was writing that, whilst he could not say that puerperal fever and erysipelas were one and the same disease, he felt that nurses and physicians who attended patients suffering from the former should carefully wash themselves and their apparel before attending a further birth.

By 1850, Casimo Davaine and Pierre Rayer, working with the rod-shaped organism responsible for anthrax – a relatively large and easily seen bacterium – demonstrated that by taking the blood of an animal suffering from the disease and injecting it into healthy sheep the disease could be reproduced, and that following the death of the animal the same bacterium could be found in its blood.

However, despite the scientific evidence accumulating throughout the seventeenth and most of the eighteenth centuries, a philosophical battle raged between those who believed that diseases were definitely contagious, and those who attributed epidemic illnesses to causes such as environmental change and internal bodily derangements. On the side of the anti-contagionists was the evidence that quarantine was not always convincingly

1

successful, that an epidemic such as yellow fever was often abruptly terminated by a change in the weather, and that other, completely different causes of disease had been proved in a number of cases, such as the dietary deficiency of scurvy. That epidemics were most prevalent in slums was interpreted by the anti-contagionists as evidence that environmental causes, rather than living creatures, were the prime instigators of disease.

Despite such arguments, in practical terms a minority of physicians had begun to recognize the relationship between relative cleanliness and a reduction in the incidence of certain fatal diseases. In the United Kingdom, Ireland and the United States, it had been recognized that a 'clean' obstetrician resulted in a reduction in the number of cases of puerperal fever in the lying-in wards, but the most famous figure in this regard was the Viennese obstetrician, Semmelweis (1818–65) who, by statistical methods, proved the contagious nature of postpartum infection and, by the use of a strict regime of hand washing and soaking the hands in chlorinated lime solution, lowered the incidence of obstetrical deaths in his wards from 18 % to about 1 %. Despite this remarkable achievement, Semmelweis's work was ignored and denigrated. His end was bitter; in the early part of the nineteenth century he was committed to an asylum and died of septicaemia.

In 1827 Joseph Lister was born. He was to become a surgeon in Edinburgh and Glasgow and later in London. Lister's seminal observation concerned the healing of fractures; he recognized that, whilst simple fractures in which the skin remained intact usually healed without complications, when the skin was broken, thus exposing the bony fragments, pus often formed with the result that delayed union or death followed. He drew the conclusion that some invisible particles, which he called 'disease dust', floating in the air were responsible.

At this point, the work of Pasteur was brought to his attention and Lister quickly realized the connection between his own observations on wounds and the microscopic bacteria which Pasteur had shown were responsible for fermentation.

Lister now introduced his carbolic acid spray, the general concept being that the organisms responsible for infection of a wound should be killed before they could enter the wound by means of a spray of carbolic acid held in close proximity to the wound or operative incision. Lister's results in 11 cases were written up in a paper in the Lancet in 1867, in which he gave full recognition to the work of Pasteur. As with Semmelweis, so Lister faced considerable opposition to his theories not only in the United Kingdom but also in the United States, although his ideas were rapidly adopted on the continent by the great surgeons of the day, including Volkmann, Langenbeck and others. Thus the use of antiseptic surgery spread.

And yet by 1887 Lister had abandoned the spray, reasoning that as the droplets of carbolic acid spread out from the nozzle of the spray so contact between the acid and the bacteria might be so reduced as to render the system useless. Lister compensated for the absence of the spray by antiseptic washings and irrigation, surrounding the site of the operation with widespread towels rung out in antiseptics.

In parallel with the work of Lister went the work of other British surgeons such as Lawson Tait who, whilst not believing in Lister's antiseptic surgery, nevertheless observed strict rules of cleanliness and who could therefore be regarded as one of the innovators of aseptic surgery – the exclusion of germs from the wound – as opposed to antiseptic surgery – the killing of germs prior to or after they have entered the wound.

2 Sterilization

INTRODUCTION

One of the chief components of aseptic surgery is the use of sterilization to destroy all forms of living organisms which by entering a wound may result in local infection or even death of the individual. Such organisms may be present in the environment in which the operation is being performed, be carried by inanimate objects, such as the instruments, swabs, packs and other materials used during the course of the operation, or by the surgeon and his operating team.

In this section, interest is focused on the sterilization of the instruments and accessories rather than the operating team and the environment.

The term sterility is absolute, implying the death of every pathogen since even a small fraction of the original number could, under suitable circumstances, give rise to a new and potentially harmful population.

As surgery has increased in scope and complexity, consideration has had to be given not only to the sterilization of instruments, swabs and drapes, but also to the various materials and objects which may be left in situ for as long as the patient survives. Thus, methods have been explored to find the most acceptable manner of sterilizing, for example, prosthetic materials used in vascular and orthopaedic surgery, cardiac pacemakers and their associated leads and heart valves.

In all cases in which specialized materials are being used, it is self evident that whatever sterilizing agent is used to achieve sterility it must not harm the material undergoing sterilization.

The following methods have been used:

1. Exposure to heat
2. Filtration

3. Ionizing radiation
4. Chemical agents.

HEAT

Heat can be used in a dry or moist form.

The application of dry heat in the surgical field is limited to the use of a hot air oven which consists of a metal chamber in which, by means of gas or electrical elements, temperatures of 160°C can be achieved. After one hour at such temperatures, sterilization is complete. Such a method can be used for the sterilization of metal instruments or bowls. In the past, infra-red rays were used for the sterilization of glass syringes, which were exposed to temperatures of 180°C. However, in the highly industrialized countries of the West, glass syringes have now been discarded and replaced by disposable plastics and, because of the fear of AIDS, needles are no longer cleaned after use but discarded. Red heat is still used by the bacteriologist to sterilize the platinum wire used to innoculate culture media with suspected materials.

Moist heat

Whilst dry heat kills by charring the cell constituents, moist heat kills organisms by coagulation and denaturization of their proteins. The simplest form of moist heat used is boiling water: boiling at 100°C for 5–10 minutes is sufficient to kill all non-sporing and many, though not all, sporing organisms. Until the early 1950's, no surgical ward was considered completely equipped or efficient without a simple form of sterilizer using boiling water to treat instruments to be used for wound dressings. In general, simple 'boiling' sterilizers have now been displaced by sterile disposable instruments and syringes. A practical disadvantage of boiling is that the instruments treated in this manner remain wet.

A second method known as 'Tyndallization', is now obsolete. It involved the exposure of objects to steam at 100°C for 30 minutes on three successive days. The first exposure killed all vegetative organisms present but had little effect on spores. These germinated overnight and were supposedly killed on the second exposure. The third steaming was a precautionary measure. However, since spores germinate erratically, the method is basically unreliable.

THE AUTOCLAVE

Such simple methods have now been replaced by the use of the autoclave, in which pressurized steam is used as a means of sterilization.

Water at atmospheric pressure boils at 100°C, but when pressure is exerted upon its surface the boiling point rises and the temperature of the steam rises in parallel with the water temperature. Furthermore, as the steam condenses, energy is released in the form of latent heat to create temperatures of 121–135°C, making pressurized steam an extremely effective agent. However, to be effective, the steam must be:

1. Dry – not carrying suspended droplets of water, since water interferes with the removal of air and the drying of the load.
2. Not superheated, since this interferes with penetration and condensation.
3. Free from air, since an admixture of air when the autoclave is operating decreases the chamber temperature at the selected pressure.

Two basic types of autoclave are in use. In both, the inner chamber containing the material to be sterilized is surrounded by an outer jacket into which steam, and therefore heat, can be introduced, thus preheating the sterilizing chamber and so reducing the possibility of condensation.

Downward (gravity) displacement autoclave. The earlier of the two types of autoclave in use is the 'downward displacement' or 'gravity displacement autoclave', currently used for the sterilization of instrument trays and instruments, but not theatre linen.

In this type, the jacket is heated and the load to be sterilized is introduced into the chamber, the articles being arranged loosely to allow the free circulation of steam and the displacement of air. The door of the autoclave is then closed and steam introduced into the chamber through a baffle high in the back of the chamber. The steam tends to float as a layer above the cooler, denser air, but as more steam is introduced the air is displaced downwards, across the articles of the load and out through a discharge channel at the bottom of the chamber. The water of condensation formed on the cool load also drains through this channel, which is controlled by a thermostatic steam trap. The channel remains open until all the condensate and air have passed through, after which, with an internal temperature of 121°C, the trap automatically closes.

A holding period of 12 minutes now elapses, a period timed to start when the thermometer in the discharge channel first shows the temperature to be 121°C. Should the temperature drop – possibly because air is displaced from the load if this is porous – and a condensate form, this collects above the trap; with the consequent drop in temperature, the trap automatically opens, the condensate drains away, the trap closes, the temperature rises once again and the holding period is automatically prolonged. The holding period is succeeded by a cooling or drying period. Thus the cycle of this type of autoclave passes through four phases:

1. The heating-up and air displacement period.
2. The holding period – normally not less than 12 minutes at 121 °C.
3. A safety period of half the sterilizing time.
4. The cooling period.

Great care should be taken not to open this type of autoclave until the internal pressure has fallen to that of the atmosphere, otherwise severe scalds may be sustained.

High pre-vacuum autoclave. The second, and more modern, type of autoclave which is now found in most central sterile supply departments is the 'high pre-vacuum autoclave.' In this type, an electrically driven pump is used to evacuate 98% of the air from the inner chamber prior to the admission of steam. This enables the steam to penetrate rapidly and heat up all parts of the load, thus producing a uniform sterilizing temperature. This makes it possible to employ higher sterilizing temperatures for a shorter time using steam temperatures of 135°C for only three minutes at 30 lb/ in^2 pressure. The load is then dried by drawing a second vacuum after which the vacuum is broken by admission of air through a filter. The normal cycle of such an autoclave therefore consists of the following:

1. The heating period, during which the outer jacket is heated.
2. The evacuation time, during which 98% of the air in the sterilizing chamber is removed.
3. The holding period, consisting of the sterilizing time.
4. A safety period, normally about one-half the sterilization time.
5. The drying time.
6. The cooling period.

This method is not suitable for bottled fluids, but is extremely useful for pre-packed trays of instruments, swabs and dressings.

Testing autoclave efficiency

Because adequate sterilization is the corner stone upon which all modern surgical techniques depend, it is essential that the performance of autoclaves in use are continously monitored.

The tests required to ensure that autoclaves or hot air sterilizers are working effectively are described in Hospital Technical Memorandum No. 10. The tests described should be carried out regularly, and the results should be available for inspection.

1. The master temperature recording (MTR). This is a graphic chart produced when the autoclave is properly commissioned against a multi-lead thermocouple recorder. The MTR should be displayed near the autoclave so as to be readily available, and all subsequent charts checked against it. If the cycle chart is not identical to the MTR, sterility cannot be guaranteed.

2. Bowie-Dick test. First described by Bowie and others in 1963 in the Lancet, this test is designed to assess whether adequate heat penetration of the load has been achieved. A standard test pack is made up of 36 Huckback Towels, 36" x 24" BSS 1781, T15 which are folded eight times before being placed in a cuboid container. In the centre are placed two strips of paper in the form of a St. Andrew's Cross of M.M.M.No. 1222 Autoclave tape, which is widely used for sealing bundles, and will indicate the effectiveness of the steam sterilizing process. If all the air has been removed from the chamber, the steam will penetrate the load rapidly and the tape will show uniform change. If all the air has not been removed, when steam is admitted the air will be forced into the centre of the pack where it will form a bubble. When the load is removed, the colour of the tape in the region of the bubble will be paler than elsewhere because of the lower central temperature, and this will be evident at the end of the 'run'. For this test, the holding time should not exceed $3\frac{1}{2}$ minutes when a temperature of 134°C is being used.

This test is only used for high-vacuum machines and not for downward displacement sterilizers.

FILTRATION

The most commonly used filters for the removal of bacteria from fluids are membrane filters made of cellulose acetate of varying pore size. To exclude bacteria a pore size of less than 0.25 μm is required. To remove bacteria from air entering the operating theatre, either 'paper absolute filters' are used which remove 99% of particles between 0.1 μm and 0.5 μm in diameter, or the air can be filtered by electrostatic precipitation.

IONIZING RADIATION

This method of sterilization is normally used commercially since the necessary apparatus is too expensive for general application. All ionizing irradiation, electrons, X-rays and gamma-rays in sufficient doses are effective in killing living tissue by inducing damage to DNA. Bacterial species vary in their sensitivity, and spores are more resistant than vegetative forms. Normally sterilization by radiation is performed using high-speed electrons produced by a linear accelerator, or using an isotope source such as Cobalt 60. This method is particularly useful for the sterilization of surgical sutures, gloves, various types of catheter, dressings and plastic protheses.

CHEMICAL AGENTS

Chemical agents for use in the environment are not strictly sterilizing agents. They should be called disinfectants or antiseptics, – terms which indicate that the agent may kill or inhibit many microorganisms without implying that they can be relied upon to kill all microorganisms and spores.

There is no clear-cut distinction between a disinfectant and an antiseptic. Some agents are disinfectants at high concentrations and antiseptics at low ones. Strong disinfectants are relatively toxic substances, rapidly killing vegetative forms of pathogenic organisms though they are often ineffective against spores. They are too poisonous or irritant to be applied to human tissues and are therefore only suitable for use on inanimate objects. Mild disinfectants, otherwise classified as antiseptics, are sufficiently bland and non-toxic for superficial application to living tissues, such as intact mucous membranes, broken skin or the interior of a wound. An antiseptic may kill a microorganism or may merely prevent its further growth – the 'bacteriostatic effect'.

The disinfectants currently available are divisible into the following groups:

1. Phenols, alcohols, aldehydes and related compounds.
2. Halogens.

3. Dyes.
4. Surface active agents.
5. Metals.
6. Derivatives of furan.
7. Amidines and guanidines.
8. Derivatives of quinoline and isoquinoline.

The probable antimicrobial effect of the majority of disinfectants is by denaturing or altering proteins or lipids in the cytoplasmic membrane. Some interfere with the energy-yielding systems within the cells, and yet others inhibit specific steps in biosynthetic pathways. Mercurial salts combine with sulphydryl groups, and antibacterial dyes combine with nucleic acids. Materials such as proflavine, a heterotrycyclic dye, combines with the guanine bases of nucleic acid: when exposed to fluorescent light, the dye absorbs energy causing single strand breaks by excision of guanine, an effect referred to as a 'photodynamic action'.

Factors controlling the action of disinfectants include:

1. Concentration.
2. Duration of contact with the pathogen.
3. Temperature, assuming that the temperature is within the limits of the thermostability of the disinfectant.
4. pH.
5. Presence of organic matter.

The three main purposes for which disinfectants are used are:

1. To decontaminate objects before their disposal or re-use.
2. The reduction of microbial contamination of an inanimate environment, e.g. baths, wash basins and toilets.
3. Disinfection of the skin of the hands and operating site.

Phenols

One of the most powerful disinfectants is phenol, carbolic acid. Phenol is too irritant to be allowed to come into contact with the skin. The chief use of its derivatives, such as Lysol (an alkylphenol obtained from the distillation of tar) is for the decontamination of bathrooms and hospital floors. Solutions of 0.3–0.65 cresol will kill the majority of common pathogens within ten minutes, but spores require higher concentrations for longer periods. Cresols have the advantage of not being quenched by organic materials. Dettol, a chlorinated xylenol is a widely used disinfectant and antiseptic for domestic purposes. It is not irritant but it is inactive against *Pseudomonas pyocyanea*.

Alcohols

Ethyl alcohol is used for rapid skin disinfection. A 70% solution in water will coagulate all proteins and kill bacteria and some viruses, but it does not readily penetrate organic matter.

Halogens

Chlorine, iodine and compounds which release chlorine, such as sodium hypochlorite, are lethal to bacteria, viruses, fungi and spores; they act by oxidising SH groups. The chief disadvantage of halogens is their susceptibility to quenching by organic matter, thus limiting their clinical application. Iodine, as a 2% solution in isopropyl alcohol, is an excellent skin disinfectant but must not be used if the skin surface is breached or the individual is known to suffer from iodine sensitivity. Iodophors are solutions of iodine in a non-ionic surface active detergent. Betadine®, a preparation in common use, contains 0.75% available iodine.

Metallic salts

Salts of mercury, silver and copper, once in common use in surgical practice, are little used today. The exception is thiomercal B.P. (Merthiolate®) which is used for the preservation of biological products.

Dyes

Dyes such as gentian violet and brilliant green are active against some Gram-positive organisms and are relatively non-toxic. Their profound disadvantage is their staining property and they are rarely used at the present time. However, the acridine dyes, such as proflavine, which is active against both Gram-positive and Gram-negative organisms, are still in common use for local application to burns and abrasions.

3 The operating theatre and its team

THE OPERATING THEATRE

In 1962, the Medical Research Council, in considering the design of operating theatre complexes, recommended six basic requirements which they considered necessary if infection from this source was to be eliminated:

1. The separation of the theatre complex from the general traffic and air movement of the hospital.
2. A sequence within the complex of increasingly clean zones from the entrance onwards into the operating room itself.
3. The ability of staff to move from one 'clean' area to another wihout passing through 'dirty' areas.
4. The removal of 'unclean' materials from the suite without passing through clean areas.
5. An airflow from clean to less clean areas.
6. Heating and ventilation to ensure a safe and comfortable environment for the patients and staff.

In hospitals built in the years immediately following the MRC recommendations, many theatre complexes were designed and built incorporating these six requirements. Among the chief results were the complete separation of the 'clean' from the 'dirty' areas by means of the 'two corridor' system, and the complete isolation of the theatre suite from facilities essential to its efficient function. Both of these practices have since been abandoned. Further, the introduction of plastic bags which can be sealed has meant that, in a disciplined environment, materials can be 'bagged' and removed with little danger of contaminating the theatre environment.

It is now considered that the theatre complex should incorporate a recovery area, which should be sited close to an intensive care unit. It is also recognized that the operation of the theatre complex will be facilitated, and other departments benefit, if it is easily accessible to the accident and emergency, X-ray, pathology and the central sterile supply departments.

In addition, it should be appreciated that an operating theatre room does not stand in perfect isolation. Although the 40 m^2 normally regarded as sufficient in area for most operations represents the focal point of the surgeons activities and thoughts, provision must be made adjacent to the theatre for:

1. Scrubbing and gowning.
2. The accomodation of the patient in an anaesthetic room which is large enough to contain the patient, the anaesthetist and his team and their apparatus.
3. A preparation room in which sterile trolleys can be laid up by the 'scrub nurse' and her assistant.

Peripheral to these facilities there must also be utility rooms, changing rooms and rest rooms for all grades of staff.

Nevertheless, the necessity to isolate the operating room itself from the surrounding areas remains paramount. The most essential service in this respect is to provide effective ventilation, since it has been repeatedly shown that the reduction of the bacterial count within a theatre is proportional to the volume of air supplied. The objectives of adequate ventilation are:

1. To prevent the ingress of bacteria from outside corridors or the external environment.
2. To remove airborne bacteria released into the theatre environment.
3. To provide a working temperature suitable for both the staff and the patient.
4. To regulate the humidity and thus reduce the danger of electrostatic sparks.

Any ventilation system must counteract the effects of convection, the movement of personnel and, in particular, the turbulence consequent upon opening/closing doors.

To fulfill these requirements the ventilation plant normally includes filters with a minimum arrestance of 85% when tested in accordance with British Standard 6540, although in areas of high atmospheric pollution higher standards of filtration may be justified to reduce staining of the interior finishes. If possible, the air handling plant should be sited as remotely as possible from sources of contamination, and protected from adverse weather conditions.

In the older, conventional theatres, ventilation was provided by ceiling-mounted air diffusers. The air volume supplied did not usually exceed $1.0 \ m^3/s$, and the air introduced into the theatre escaped by way of vents situated just above floor level, and through any gaps in the doors.

Other methods of ventilation have been tried, including the introduction of air from high on the side walls – so-called 'lateral' supply – although this method has gained little popularity since projected at the operating team it tends to produce a chilling effect.

More recently still has been the introduction of ultraclean ventilation systems, in which a high flow of filtered air is directed vertically downwards leaving the area of the theatre in which the operation is being carried out virtually free from contamination. Because the flow is vertical, the possibility that the operating team will introduce bacteria into the airstream is considerably reduced. Theatre lighting, if this system is introduced, has to be carefully positioned so as not to interrupt the air stream.

In some types of surgery, additional protection against contamination is obtained by the use of body exhaust suits fitted with head pieces, the latter having become popular with the orthopaedic surgeons engaged in joint replacement operations.

In addition to countering bacterial hazards, gas scavenging systems are now mandatory in all operating systems.

Routine tests of the theatre environment include temperature recordings – the ideal ambient temperature being 21°C (72°F) – and hygrometer readings to measure the relative humidity, which should not be allowed to fall below 55%.

Routine bacteriological examination of the theatre is not required unless the operating theatre has been closed for some time or some work has been performed on its internal structure. After the list is finished all that is needed is to wash the walls and floor with a detergent such as HOSPEC. If , however, a patient suffering from hepatitis B has been in the theatre, the floor should be washed with 10% hypochlorite (Chloros 10 000 p.p.m.) and all surfaces damp dusted with 1% hypochlorite, 1 000 p.p.m. The surgeon should take the additional precaution of wearing goggles. Similarly, if a patient suffering from HIV infection has passed through the theatre the same schedule should be observed, with the additional precaution that any spillage on the floor should be immediately dealt with by an application of glutaraldehyde.

SCRUB TECHNIQUE FOR THE SURGEON AND THE OPERATING TEAM

The taps in the area reserved for scrubbing are turned on and the temperature of the water is adjusted. The hands and forearms are moistened and a liberal quantity of 4% chlorhexidine BP or betadine 7.5 w/v is applied, after which the team wash up to the elbows for one minute.

Chlorhexidine belongs to the amidine and guanidine group and is a bisguanidine active against a wide range of Gram-positive and negative organisms. Chlorhexidine is, however, inhibited by the presence of blood. Its action is probably mediated by reacting with the cytoplasmic membrane, disorganizing it and destroying its function. It will inactivate *Staphylococcus aureus* in dilutions as low as 0.5 p.p.m. Betadine (povidone-iodine) is an iodophor, a complex of iodine and a 'solubilizer'. Iodine used in this fashion can be left on the skin long enough to remove most spores. Unfortunately, this being an iodine-containing preparation, some members of the team may be sensitive to it. In various critical reviews, 4% chlorhexidine appears to be the most effective material to use.

Following the one-minute wash, a sterile brush is now obtained, more lotion is applied and the fingernails of each hand are scrubbed for about one minute. The brush is then discarded, more lotion is supplied and the hands thoroughly washed over a period of approximately two minutes. The hands are then rinsed and water allowed to drain off at the elbows, after which they can be dried on a sterile towel.

PREPARATION OF THE PATIENT'S SKIN

Since a rapid reduction in skin flora is required in the preoperative preparation of the skin site, a quick-acting antiseptic is necessary. A variety of compounds are available including 10% aqueous betadine, 1% iodine in alcohol and 0.5% chlorhexidine in 70% alcohol. In some cases the surgeon demands that the skin preparation is commenced on the day prior to the operation, for which purpose iodine in alcohol, or hexachlorophane liquid soap, are satisfactory.

Despite the use of the agents described, it must be emphasized that sterility is not an absolute concept in practice. Lowbury and his co-workers, who have performed much work on this subject, showed that the mean estimated reduction of skin flora was

99.98%. In other words, with a variety of agents absolute sterility was not obtained by the surgeon and, as far as the patient's skin was concerned, treatment was even less effective. In spite of this, in the majority of patients this massive reduction of the bacterial flora renders the operation safe. However, a variety of factors may lead to increasing rates of infection in clean surgical wounds: prominent among these are an operation of long duration leading to excessive sweating, pricking of gloves, which occurs in about 30% of operations, contamination of the skin by blood, and obesity.

4 The healing wound

The manner in which wounds heal is classically divided into:

1. Healing by primary intention, when the wound is closed by sutures and heals without complications.
2. Healing by secondary intention, when the wound is left open or becomes so because of some complication.

The essential differences between healing by primary and secondary intention are that in the latter not only is extensive epithelialization necessary but considerable quantities of connective tissue are also formed, this last leading, as it matures, to the contraction of the wound.

FACTORS AFFECTING WOUND HEALING

The aim of the surgeon after making an incision is to lay the foundations for healing by primary intention. Infection delays healing – hence the need for the precautions discussed in Chapters 2 and 3. The incision, involving not only the skin but also aponeuroses and in some cases muscle, is drawn together by sutures of various types. Assuming that the wound does not become infected, healing by primary intention will be achieved so long as the patient is relatively healthy prior to his or her operation.

Delay in healing may occur in the debilitated, malnourished individual who has lost some 20% of bodyweight prior to the operation. The wound has been described as a parasite taking precedence over all other functions, but this is only natural since without effective healing an individual's life is at risk. Some of the specific factors affecting wound healing are discussed below.

Vitamin C

Lack of vitamin C results in slow healing, absence of healing or even in the breakdown of wounds already healed. This is due to interference with collagen formation in the endoplasmic reticulum of the fibroblast, the collagen being synthesized from the amino acids, glycine, proline and hydroxyproline. Initially, neither hydroxyproline nor hydroxyglycine are incorporated directly into the collagen molecule. Instead, a proline-rich collagen precursor known as protocollagen is formed. Hydroxylation then occurs under the influence of protocollagen hydroxylase, and it is at this stage that lack of vitamin C plays its part. In its absence, the incompletely synthesized collagen cannot be excreted from the fibroblasts and merely accumulates within the endoplasmic reticulum.

Oxygen

Wounds made in tissues in which there is a lack of oxygen due to circulatory deficiency heal more slowly than do wounds in normal tissues. Hence, the wound of an amputation stump may be slow to heal or may readily break down after the sutures are removed, as may wounds made in tissues which have been previously irradiated. Experimental evidence has shown that fibroblastic activity is maximal up to 50–80 μm away from the nearest normally perfused capillary, at which point the Po_2 level is between 10 and 20 mmHg (1.3–2.6 kPa). At lower oxygen tensions fibroblastic activity fails. Macrophages, an important element in wound healing, require less oxygen than do fibroblasts and are found at the free edge of growing granulation tissue where they are still able to ingest bacteria. However, their ability to kill bacteria is in some doubt since the killing mechanism is mediated by the oxygen-dependent peroxidase system.

Zinc

Although it can be shown in an experimental animal that zinc, an important component of many enzyme systems, will promote the healing of thermal burns, the evidence in humans is more tenuous. However, it has been shown by some workers that the administration of zinc hastens the healing of open wounds produced by the excision of pilonidal sinuses, possibly by stimulating the biosynthesis of collagen.

Glucocorticoids

The administration of glucocorticoids delays wound healing by causing defects in collagen synthesis, as also do the antimitotic drugs.

Infection

The commonest cause of delayed healing in an incised wound is without doubt infection. An incised wound carefully closed, even when adequate haemostasis is achieved, has no resistance to bacteria during the first six hours. Thereafter it becomes increasingly difficult to infect the wound until, at five days, it is as resistant to infection as the surrounding skin. When infection occurs, collagenolytic activity is greatly increased.

HEALING BY PRIMARY INTENTION

The healing of a clean incised wound passes through the following stages.

1. Haematoma formation

However effective haemostasis and the suturing of a wound may be, some blood still collects between the sides of the incision resulting in the formation of a fibrin-rich haematoma.

2. Epithelialization

Within hours of injury the epithelial cells from the adjacent epidermis migrate into the wound and insinuate themselves between the inert dermis and the haematoma. Within 24 hours in a well-approximated wound, a continuous layer of epidermal cells covers the surface, although this will not be apparent to the naked eye since this layer is covered by a crust of dried blood. Within the next 24–48 hours, the epidermal cells invade the space where connective tissue will eventually develop, forming an epithelial spur pointing downwards into the underlying dermis. The migrating cells of the epidermis do not divide; the mitotic activity leading to this cellular migration takes place in the basal cells a short distance from the edge of the wound, possibly due to a decline in the area of a wound-specific inhibitory factor called a chalone.

3. Demolition phase

Monocytes and macrophages migrate into the wound to remove the clot and cellular debris, reaching their most numerous within 2–3 days.

4. Organization

On or about the third day, the wound area is invaded by capillary buds and fibroblasts. This is the granulation tissue so much more prominent in a wound healing by secondary intention. As soon as the fibroblasts appear, collagen begins to form and slowly matures. When normal collagen is examined by polarized light, it stands out as a birefringent material. In a recent wound the collagen does not exhibit this quality, indicating a failure of organization at the molecular or small fibril level which takes about six months to rectify. However, the normal arrangement of collagen, with its well-organized bundles, never occurs; in a wound, the newly formed collagen coalesces to form large irregular masses which are never remodelled. Although the active laying down of collagen proceeds rapidly, collagenase is also released when the wound is made. The formation of granulation tissue appears to prevent excessive epithelial migration into the wound, and the epithelial cells forming the spur or lining the tracks made by suture material degenerate to be replaced by granulation tissue. Only the surface cells persist, and these divide and differentiate to reform the multi-layered epidermis.

From the surgeon's viewpoint, the strength of the healing wound is its most important property.

In the first few days, the integrity of the wound is wholly dependent upon the sutures which have been inserted. It is during this period, variously called the lag phase, demolition phase or preparation phase, that the devitalized tissues are removed. However, as soon as the fibroblasts begin to lay down collagen, the ability of the wound to resist rupture increases rapidly although recent investigation has shown that even after six months the strength of the wound rarely exceeds 70% of the norm. Fortunately, such is the overcompensation that this is more than sufficient to meet the stresses normally imposed.

HEALING BY SECONDARY INTENTION

The difference between healing by secondary, as opposed to primary intention, is quantitative rather than qualitative. In a wound which is open, healing must take place from the base upwards and from the edges inwards. An appropriate model would be the wound caused by a full thickness burn or scald. In such a wound, the importance of the contraction which takes place in helping to diminish the area of epithelialization is readily apparent; this occurs to the greatest extent in wounds situated where the skin is only loosely attached to the underlying tissues.

WOUNDS OF THE GASTROINTESTINAL TRACT

Healing of wounds of the stomach and small intestine proceeds without incident in the vast majority of cases, but anastomoses made in the oesophagus or colon heal much less reliably. This is primarily because their blood supply is relatively poor and they possess less collagen prior to injury than either the stomach or the small bowel. Furthermore, bacterial contamination is greater in the oesophagus and colon. Because of this, greater quantities of collagen undergo lysis, in a situation in which this material is already in short supply, with the result that the suture line tends to be weak and may give way when exposed to an increase in intraluminal pressure.

It is common practice to restore the continuity of bowel in two layers; the first consists of an interrupted layer including the seromuscular layer; and the second, inner, layer consists of a continous stitch which includes the whole thickness of the bowel wall. Several studies have suggested that a two-layer anastomosis possesses little advantage over the simpler one-layer technique, but the majority of surgeons continue to use the two-layer technique and, even when employing stapling devices, continue to reinforce such an anastomosis with a series of interrupted sutures.

5 Ligatures and sutures

Because the majority of vessels encountered by the surgeon in the course of an operation are controlled by ligatures, and because the strength of a wound or anastomosis depends, at least initially, on the presence of sutures, it is necessary for the surgeon to have some knowledge of the materials which are available.

In general terms, both ligatures and sutures are one of two types: absorbable or non-absorbable. Absorbable materials are digested and, in the majority of patients, leave no trace of their presence after healing of the wound is complete. However, in a minority of patients, because of the various processes to which natural materials are subjected and the varying reactions of an individual's tissues, small fragments of so-called absorbable materials may still be found embedded in the tissues many months or even years later, acting as foreign bodies and providing no support whatsoever.

Absorbable ligatures and sutures include natural materials, such as catgut, collagen and living sutures such as are derived from aponeuroses, and the synthetic material, polyglycolic acid.

The non-absorbable ligatures and sutures again consist of natural and synthetic materials, and also metals which can be formed into sutures or clips. The naturally-occurring non-absorbable materials, now rarely used, include silk in various forms, linen and cotton. Among the synthetic materials available are the polyamides, polyesters and the polylectons.

NATURALLY-OCCURRING ABSORBABLE MATERIALS

Catgut

For many years, the only absorbable material available for the ligature of vessels and the construction of intestinal anastomoses was catgut. Most was obtained from the upper third of the small bowel of New Zealand sheep. The appropriate segment of gut was removed, mechanically cleansed and the 'caseings' frozen for transport to the manufacturer. After arrival, they were thawed, split into three or four ribbons and then scraped to remove the muscle, mucosa and fatty tissue. What is left is essentially a pure collagen strip formed of the submucosal layer. According to the diameter of the product required, two or more ribbons are spun together into strands before drying under tension and the surface is then polished. The product at this stage is plain catgut. This is normally absorbed within 5–10 days when buried in muscle tissue, or in a fraction of this time when used to approximate the peritoneum or a serous membrane.

Since the latter period is normally judged too short for consolidation, 'plain' catgut is hardened by immersing it in salts of chromium which cause the collagen to harden and thus be less readily absorbed. Although chromic catgut is naturally colourless, a dye is added to the preparation so that chromised catgut assumes a deep brown colour. The degree to which hardening occurs is a function of the duration of exposure to the chromic salts. Normally, chromic catgut will persist in the tissues for some 15–20 days, and somewhat less in the peritoneum. Each strand is graded for size, the smallest size (using the old scale, with which the majority of surgeons remain familiar) is 6/0 and the largest 2. As the diameter increases, so too does the tensile strength and the load required to break the fibre.

After division of the strands into lengths, each piece is wound onto a card or plastic former. After covering with a suitable material the catgut is sealed into a foil pack containing a minimum amount of purified methylated spirit after which it is sterilized by irradiation. In general terms, the size and type of catgut used is determined by surgical preference, some surgeons ligating all vessels with plain catgut and others using all chromic gut. Whilst smaller sizes are required for ligating vessels and for anastomoses, larger-diameter fibres are required to close the peritoneum; because of its rapid absorption, plain catgut is never used for this purpose.

Living suture material

Tissue sutures can be obtained from the patient. Although fashionable some decades ago they are rarely used today. The commonest operation in which living tissue was used was for the repair of large inguinal or recurrent herniae by the method described by Gallie. Using this method, a long strand of tensor fascia lata was taken from the outer aspect of the thigh and the wound closed. Then, after securing the strip to a large but cumbersome needle known as a Gallie's needle, the fascial strip was used to suture the conjoint tendon to the inguinal ligament. The majority of surgeons obtained the fascial strip by making a long longitudinal skin incision in the thigh, removing the fascia with great care, making sure not to cut across its fibres.

Collagen tape

Manufactured by Ethicon and supplied in lengths 60 cm long and 3 mm in width, collagen tape can be used as a substitute for autologous and homologous fascia in various operations, especially repair of lacerations of the liver.

SYNTHETIC ABSORBABLE MATERIALS

The number of synthetic materials increases yearly and this section will therefore discuss merely a small selection of those that can be used.

The first absorbable synthetic material to be used in surgery was the synthetic polymer of glycolic acid known commercially as Dexon and introduced by Davis and Geck in 1970. In contrast to catgut and collagen, which are digested by proteolytic enzymes, Dexon is absorbed by hydrolysis. The material is developed by extrusion of fine strands which are then braided to form a uniform gauge thread varying in size from 6/0 to 1. Complete resorption takes place at between 60 and 90 days. Dexon is extremely inert, fray-resistant and the knot does not tend to slip; this last can be a disadvantage since after making the first knot of the ligature the suture will not 'snug' down under an additional throw.

Additional synthetic absorbable sutures have rapidly been developed; these include;

1. *Polyglactin 910 (Coated Vicryl)*. This is a braided suture coated so that it runs easily through the tissues. It is twice as strong as catgut on implantation and loses only half its strength in the first 14 days. It is absorbed by hydrolysis.
2. *Polydioxanone*. This is a monofilamentous suture which loses only 30% of its strength over the first 28 days.

NATURALLY-OCCURRING NON-ABSORBABLE MATERIALS

Natural materials, such as silk, linen and cotton, were extensively used in the past but have now been largely superseded. All are multifilamentous and are supplied in a variety of sizes with variable breaking loads according to the diameter.

SYNTHETIC NON-ABSORBABLE MATERIALS

Nylon

The first plastic material introduced into surgical use during the Second World War was the polyamide known as nylon. It is available as a monofilamentous or multifilamentous thread. Monofilamentous nylon, usually blue in colour, is supplied in a variety of sizes and lengths. Being an inert monofilamentous material, it can be used in the presence of infection. Its disadvantage is that slight slippage of the knot may occur, making the thicker strands more difficult to use.

Braided nylon is similar in character to braided silk and is supplied between 4/0 and 4.

Terylene

This polyester fibre is better known under its trade name, Dacron, and is available as a white or blue thread. Seldom used as a suture material, Dacron has found its chief niche when woven into a vascular prothesis and it is also used in a flat woven form to repair massive defects in the abdominal wall.

Polyolefins

Polybutester. This is available as a blue monofilamentous suture supplied by Davies and Geck under the trade name of Norafil. It produces a minimal foreign body reaction and does not easily slip. It can be supplied as an atraumatic suture, when it is chiefly used in plastic and vascular surgery.

Polypropylene. Marketed under the name of Prolene or Miraline by Ethicon, this is an extremely inert monofilamentous fibre. It is available in a wide range of fibre sizes varying from 10/0 to 2. It's knot-holding capacity is superior to that of other synthetic suture materials. Coated with PTFE it becomes known as Tricon, which is extensively used in open heart surgery for valve replacement.

Metallic wires

Three metals have been used; stainless steel, the alloy, tantalum, and silver. All may be obtained as single or stranded sutures, and both steel and tantalum may be braided. The use of metallic sutures is chiefly limited to orthopaedic and thoracic surgery, although in the recent past wire meshes were used for the repair of both incisional and recurrent herniae. Over the past two decades the use of metal has increased, with the various stapling devices now extensively used in gastrointestinal surgery.

SKIN CLOSURE

Skin closure can be accomplished by conventional methods using an appropriate suture material but in children, and in the scrotum in particular, an absorbable material such as Dexon can be used. A significant disadvantage of conventional closure of the skin is that each suture produces in its immediate vicinity tissue which is rigidly confined. All wounds are accompanied by an inflammatory response even in the absence of infection. Thus, the suture if tied tightly enough causes pain and, more importantly, an area in its immediate vicinity in which the blood supply is temporarily compromised, this latter causing a loss of tissue resistance and an increased susceptibility to infection. It is for this reason that adhesive micropore strips of tape, which are chemically inert and adhere to the skin, have become popular in smaller wounds; as also has the use in longer wounds of continous subcuticular stitches of a non-absorbable material which can be removed when wound healing has taken place.

6 Abdominal and thoraco-abdominal incisions

GENERAL PRINCIPLES

1. The incision chosen should give adequate exposure, e.g. the rigid adherence to the original description of McBurney for the removal of an inflamed appendix may on occasions lead to difficulty. As will be seen, the principles described by McBurney may be maintained but the actual site of the incision may need to be modified according to the physical signs found on examination of the patient.
2. Nerves should not be divided. Observation of this principle has led to the pararectal incision – described by Battle and used by previous generations of surgeons for the removal of the appendix or exploration of the pelvis – being abandoned, for the extension of this incision superiorly always resulted in the division of one or more nerves, causing the late development of an indirect hernia.
3. A wound should be protected as much as possible from contamination.
4. Careful haemostasis is required to prevent the development of haematomata which may delay healing and also add to the risk of wound infection by forming a nidus for the growth of contaminating bacteria.
5. The possible cosmetic consequences of the incision should be considered. Thus, in the neck, incisions in the skin creases should be made whenever possible.

MIDLINE AND PARAMEDIAN INCISIONS

The choice between a midline or paramedian incision for the exposure of the contents of the upper abdomen is largely a matter of individual choice. Surgeons who favour a midline incision consider that the paramedian confers no advantage in terms of long-term wound strength, and that the additional dissection required to displace the rectus abdominis laterally increases the frequency of postoperative haematomata.

Paramedian incisions

A paramedian incision can be made on either side of the midline, whichever is appropriate, and above or below the umbilicus. The wound can be extended upwards or downwards with ease.

Upper paramedian incisions

In obese individuals great care should be taken to make the skin incision well lateral to the midline, otherwise the surgeon will find himself performing a midline incision instead of a paramedian incision.

The wound is deepened through the superficial fat to the level of the anterior rectus sheath which is then divided in the line of the skin incision; alternatively, if the superficial wound has led to a more medial position over the linea alba, the superficial fat is reflected somewhat laterally. After incising the rectus sheath in a vertical direction, the medial edge is grasped by a succession of forceps, usually of the Halstead type, and the surgeon begins to dissect both the muscle and then the tendinous intersections away from the medial flap of the sheath; the lateral part of the sheath is left undisturbed. At any point in this dissection troublesome haemorrhage may be encountered which should be dealt with either by coagulation diathermy or by under-running the bleeding vessels with 2/0 catgut, whichever is more appropriate.

Once the anterior surface and the medial edge of the rectus have been released, its posterior surface is freed from the underlying posterior sheath by a mixture of blunt and sharp dissection. At the superior end of an upper paramedian incision, the muscular fibres of the transversus abdominis are normally seen running transversely towards the midline. The posterior sheath is picked up in a pair of dissecting forceps with teeth and then by artery forceps placed approximately 2 cm from the midline. The tissue held between the forceps is felt between the thumb and index finger in order to be as certain as possible that a viscus has not been accidently picked up at the same time. The posterior sheath of the rectus together with the peritoneum with which it is incorporated is then incised using a fresh scalpel, after which the incision is enlarged using scissors for the upward, and a scalpel for the downward, extension.

A minority of surgeons have advocated an incision known as the lateral paramedian incision when exploring the upper abdomen believing that this is followed by a much lower incidence of incisional herniae. To perform this incision, all that is necessary is to separate the posterior surface of the rectus abdominis from its sheath to a point just medial to its medial border. This type of incision requires some 20 minutes more time to perform and, in the author's experience, is associated with somewhat more troublesome bleeding, thereby increasing the possibility of wound haematomata and thus the possibility of infection.

In the great majority of patients the indication for surgical intervention is already known. Nevertheless, a thorough and systematic examination of the whole abdominal cavity should be carried out in order to rule out any concomitant disease.

Lower paramedian incisions

In lower paramedian incisions, used for example to perform an anterior resection of the rectum, the incision proceeds in a similar manner to the above. However, once the anterior sheath has been opened, three differences will be apparent:

1. At the lower end of the wound, the muscle fibres of the pyramidalis muscle running vertically upwards on the medial side of the rectus abdominis from the pubis will be seen.
2. The posterior sheath of the rectus at the lower limits of the incision after reflecting the rectus laterally is absent. The sheath gradually becomes thinner until it ends in the arcuate arch of Douglas which is usually situated at a point approximately midway betwen the umbilicus and the pubis.
3. The inferior epigastric artery and vein are present. These run upwards and medially towards the umbilicus and require division between ligatures.

When extending a lower paramedian incision inferiorly towards the pubis, it should be remembered that, at the lower limits of the incision, the bladder might be inadvertently injured when dividing the peritoneum.

Midline incisions

An upper midline incision is used by many surgeons for operations on the upper abdominal viscera. By an upward extension (see below) this incision can also be used to expose the lower 8–10 cm of the oesophagus. However, whilst the incision is made in the midline it should be closed by a suture (preferably of non-absorbable material) passing through the medial margins of the rectus sheath, i.e. passing through both the anterior and posterior layers. For this reason, once the linea alba has been exposed the subcutaneous tissues should be separated from its surface for a distance of up to 1.5 cm on either side of the midline.

Following this, the linea alba is incised in the midline to expose the extraperitoneal fat and peritoneum. The amount of extraperitoneal fat, particularly in an obese individual, may surprise an inexperienced operator. Vessels in this fat should be controlled by ligature rather than by diathermy because of the relative ineffectiveness of the latter when the vessels are surrounded by fat.

The upward extension of a midline incision to expose the lower oesophagus

In patients suffering from severe pulmonary disease in whom disease at the lower end of the oesophagus is present, the following incision both gives adequate exposure of the lower oesophagus and diminishes the respiratory difficulties imposed by a thoraco-abdominal incision. The midline incision is extended upwards through the skin to the level of the second intercostal space and deepened to the surface of the sternum. The loose areolar tissue on the posterior aspect of the sternum is now separated from the bone and the sternum is divided in the midline using either a Sarns saw or the older Lebsche sternal chisel, the latter being equally effective although it may be followed by more bleeding. In either case, the bleeding is controlled by applying Horsley's bone wax to the marrow of the sternum.

A sternal hook is now inserted into the upper end of the sternal incision and pulled tight, and a rib retractor is placed between the divided edges of the sternum. A clear view of the hiatus is now seen, and access to the lower part of the thoracic oesophagus is gained by dividing the central tendon of the diaphragm to which the pericardium is attached, thus exposing the lower 8–10 cm of the oesophagus.

KOCHER'S INCISION

This incision is commonly used for biliary surgery, although the incision as described by Kocher has now been considerably reduced in length due to the availability of relaxant anaesthesia. Kocher described his incision as one made two fingers' breadth below the costal margin beginning at the costal margin on the left, crossing the midline and ending laterally at the tip of the right tenth rib. As practised at the present time, the skin incision is made 2–3 cm, two fingers' breadth, below the costal margin extending from the midline to the lateral border of the rectus. After dividing the rectus sheath and the rectus muscle itself in the same direction as the skin incision, the first 2–3 cm of the flat muscles of the abdomen are also divided at the lateral extremity of the wound.

The author himself prefers a transverse incision dividing the skin in a transverse skin crease just above the level of the umbilicus, dividing the rectus sheath and the rectus muscle in the same line, and then extending the incision laterally. This incision gives adequate exposure of the extrahepatic biliary tract in the majority of patients. At the present time, an even more limited approach is being advocated by a minority of surgeons: an incision is made only 3–4 cm in length, after which the gall bladder is removed from the fundus downwards, traction on the fundus of the gallbladder revealing the extrahepatic ductal system without difficulty.

An even more recent development is laparoscopic cholecystectomy. This demands no incision as such but merely three small 1 cm wounds through which the appropriate instruments can be introduced into the abdominal cavity.

McBURNEY'S INCISION

This is the most commonly used incision for the removal of an inflamed appendix. Classically, the skin incision is made at the junction of the middle and outer thirds of the spino-umbilical line, one-third being above the line and two-thirds below. The incision is deepened through the superficial and deep fascia until the external oblique aponeurosis is reached, with its fibres passing downwards and medially towards the rectus sheath and the inguinal ligament. This aponeurosis is split in the direction of its fibres, exposing the muscle fibres of the internal oblique which pass obliquely upwards. The fibres of this muscle are then split using a suitable instrument, such as a pair of bent or flat scissors, after which the fibres of the transversus abdominis are seen running roughly along the same axis. These fibres are then separated after which the extraperitoneal fat is visible. This is separated from the underlying peritoneum which can now be opened taking the precautions previously described (p. 32).

In practice, because of its greater cosmetic acceptability, it is now more common to use a transverse skin incision made at the level of the anterior superior spine, rather than the classic oblique incision. However, a more important consideration than the cosmetic appearance of the resulting scar is that the incision should give adequate exposure of the diseased organ. To this end, although obeying the principle of muscle splitting as opposed to muscle cutting, the incision should be centred on the point of maximum tenderness as found on clinical examination of the patient. If the incision does not give adequate access to the appendix, it can be enlarged by dividing the outer edge of the rectus sheath which gives much greater exposure to the right iliac fossa. Alternatively, the flat muscles of the abdomen can be deliberately incised in an upward direction.

PFANNENSTIEL INCISION

This incision is most commonly used by abdominal surgeons for operations upon the bladder and prostate, but it is also frequently used by gynaecologists and others for operations on the uterus and its adnexa. The skin incision itself is made parallel to the suprapubic crease and below the hair line in the female. The wound is deepened until the sheath of the rectus on both sides of the midline is exposed. The fibres of the sheath are then divided transversely in the line of the skin incision, thus exposing the muscle fibres of the rectus abdominis. The sheath is then reflected in both an upward and downward direction, exposing the bellies of the rectus abdominis over a variable distance. The greater this exposure the greater the access to either the extra- or intraperitoneal tissues obtained. The loose areolar tissue between the recti is now divided, allowing their bellies to be widely separated.

The peritoneum can then be opened or, alternatively, the dissection can proceed in an extraperitoneal plane as is required, for example, to perform a retropubic prostatectomy.

THORACO-ABDOMINAL INCISION FOR EXPOSURE OF THE LOWER OESOPHAGUS AND THE UPPER END OF THE STOMACH

The patient is positioned on the table with the left side uppermost. The left arm is flexed to a right angle and held in an arm bracket attached to the table. The right leg is flexed to approximately 45° at both the hip and the knee, and the left leg is extended. A suitable bracket is used to maintain the position of the thoracic spine and a strap is used to support the buttocks.

In general, if the abdominal contents are to be exposed no greater than a two-thirds tilt is required, otherwise it becomes difficult to manipulate the upper abdominal viscera.

When seeking to expose the lower end of the oesophagus and the stomach, the line of the incision should run along the line of the eighth rib. However, the majority of patients in whom this incision is used are suffering from a carcinoma of the cardia which has spread to involve the lower end of the oesophagus; thus, the first incision should be an oblique abdominal incision passing from the midline at the level of the umbilicus upwards and outwards towards the costal cartilage of the eighth rib.

This incision is then deepened to expose the anterior rectus sheath, which is divided in the line of the incision. The rectus belly is then divided, care being taken to deal with any bleeding vessels within this muscle, after which the posterior sheath and the peritoneum are divided together.

When this exposure is used in patients suffering from malignant disease, the whole of the upper abdomen is now explored to determine the presence or absence of liver metastases, the extent of lymph node involvement and the local operability of the tumour itself.

If after due consideration a resection is deemed possible and of benefit to the patient, the skin incision is continued obliquely upwards along the line of the rib to its posterior angle. The latissimus dorsi and the fibres of the serratus anterior overlying the rib are divided and the surface of the rib exposed. The periosteum of the rib is then divided by diathermy and elevated from the superfical surface of the rib by means of a Price Thomas raspatory, from the upper border of the rib by means of a Semb raspatory, and finally from the posterior surface of the rib by the further use of the Price Thomas instrument, taking care to avoid injury to the intercostal neurovascular bundle. An incision is now made through the posterior layer of the periosteum, an incision which usually leads to the parietal pleura being opened. As this is performed so the lung, if there are no adhesions will collapse. The costal cartilage is now divided and a rib spreader of the type described by Tudor Edwards or Finochetto can be placed in the wound and the ribs spread. The abdominal and thoracic cavities are now under direct vision separated only by the diaphragm which is divided exposing both the lower oesophagus and the cardiac end of the stomach.

EXPOSURE OF THE KIDNEY

In the past the most commonly used incision to expose the kidney was by a retroperitoneal approach; an approach designed to prevent infection of the peritoneal cavity. The disadvantages of an approach through the loin are:

1. It does not allow exploration of the abdomen.
2. It precludes bilateral renal or adrenal exploration.
3. Early control of the renal vessels cannot be achieved.
   Furthermore, to reach the renal vessels the kidney must be manipulated, a grave defect when dealing with tumours of the kidney which metastasize via the blood stream.

It should also be noted that, with the exception of malignant disease, there are now relatively few indications for exploring the kidney, and if the indication is tumour then the majority of surgeons will approach the kidney transperitoneally via the abdomen.

Extraperitoneal approach

The patient is placed in the appropriate lateral position with the leg on the uppermost side extended and the inferior limb flexed. A vertical support is provided for the upper thoracic spine, and the uppermost arm is supported on a padded rest in a horizontal position flexed at the shoulder joint. A leather or canvas strap is normally applied across the patient's buttocks on a line between the iliac crest and the greater trochanter.

The position of the patient on the operating table should be such that when the table is 'broken', lateral flexion of the spine will open the costo-iliac space and so facilitate access to the kidney. A skin incision is now made over the twelfth rib, commencing immediately lateral to the outer border of the erector spinae and extending forwards for several centimetres. The skin, superficial fat and fascia are divided, exposing in the posterior extremity of the incision the fibres of latissimus dorsi, the fibres of which, arising from the thoraco-dorsal fascia, are passing in an upward direction towards the humerus. Deep to latissimus are the fibres of serratus posterior inferiores.

Division of the fibres of these muscles exposes the body of the twelfth rib, at the anterior extremity of which is the origin of the muscular fibres of the external oblique. With the rib exposed, the peritoneum over the centre of the rib is divided by diathermy and the periosteum raised from its superficial surface by raspatory. The superior border of the rib is then cleared of its periosteal attachments by a chisel-edged Semb raspatory. A Doyen rib raspatory is then inserted over the upper border of the rib, and the posterior surface and the inferior border of the rib are cleared of their attachments. At this point, care should be taken that the raspatory is in the correct plane to avoid injury to the neurovascular bundle and also the lower border of the pleura, which may be torn. The exposed rib can now be divided at its posterior angle.

The lumbosacral fascia is now divided and the external oblique, the fibres of the internal oblique and the transversus are separated by blunt dissection.

The paranephric fat is now clearly seen overlying the perirenal fascia of Gerota. The former is separated from the fascia which is then divided exposing the perinephric fat which, in the absence of serious infection, is only loosely attached to the kidney itself. The kidney can now be lifted out of the wound and dissection of the hilar structures commenced in the knowledge that the most posterior structure is the pelvis of the kidney and the most anterior the renal veins with the renal artery between the two. Each of these structures should be divided and ligated separately.

7 Wound infection

FACTORS PREDISPOSING TO WOUND INFECTION

In 1960, a report published in the Lancet by the Public Health Laboratory Service surveyed the wound infection rate in four different hospitals and found that overall some 10% of 3000 surgical wounds had become infected.

The incidence of sepsis varied between the four hospitals surveyed from 4.7% to 21.8%. At that time, it was generally believed that wounds became infected due to faulty theatre or dressing techniques, and that the chief organisms involved following 'clean' surgical wounds, such as herniotomy or mastectomy, were the aerobic staphylococci and streptococci and that following gastrointestinal operations the major offender was *Escherichia coli*. It was not until 1974 that the importance was recognized of the anaerobic *Bacteroides sp.* following gastrointestinal procedures.

The 1960 report also concluded that several factors influenced the sepsis rate, those of special importance being the age of the patient, the length of stay in hospital, the length of the incision, the duration of the operation and the use of drainage tubes. It has subsequently become apparent that other factors, excluding the number of bacteria involved, are also concerned in the development of wound infection.

These include general disorders, e.g.:

1. The individual's susceptibility to infection which, even in a normal individual, varies over several orders of magnitude.
2. More specifically inborn defects in resistance and immunity.
3. Acquired immune deficiency syndrome.
4. Hypovolaemic shock leading to poor tissue perfusion.

Among local factors are:

41

1. Trauma from over zealous retraction which causes injury to tissues in the immediate vicinity of the wound and devascularization of skin flaps.
2. Poor haemostasis.
3. The presence of foreign material, including non-absorbable ligature materials such as silk.

The chief effect of wound infection, in addition to pus formation, is delayed healing leading to the danger of dehiscence. This delay in healing can be demonstrated in the experimental animal by 'bursting' tests. These show an overall decrease in the strength of infected wounds due to depression of fibroblastic proliferation, although it has also been shown that, despite this, there is a local increase in the amount of hydroxyproline in the wound which may represent a response to the increase in collagenolytic activity.

The effects of infection following abdominal surgery are dehiscence of anastomoses followed by local or general peritonitis, fistula formation and even septicaemia, with the possibility of secondary effects such as renal, respiratory or bleeding disorders, any or all of which might lead to death. All the above complications, even if not fatal, lead inevitably to an increased length of stay in hospital.

The high rate of infection of surgical wounds noted in this and other reports prompted many surgeons to embark upon the injudicious use of antibiotics, 'covering' even 'clean' operations with long courses of these compounds. This misguided policy soon led to the emergence of resistant strains of organisms such as *Staphylococcus aureus* within the hospital environment which rapidly colonized new admissions. Worse, it resulted in an outbreak of staphylococcal pseudomembranous colitis leading to death in patients subjected to upper abdominal operations such as partial gastrectomy. As a result, there was utter condemnation of chemoprophylaxis in surgery for several years.

However, it has now become apparent that airborne infection is responsible for only 5% or less of wound infections, and that faulty dressing techniques are even less important since although the newly created wound has no resistance to infection, after a short period it is almost impossible to infect it. It has also become apparent that most wounds are infected by endogenous organisms. In clean wounds which become infected, *Staphylococcus* alone is responsible for about 50%, the coliforms alone for a further 20%

and a mixture of both in the remainder. In infections following gastrointestinal operations, the majority of bacteria responsible are anaerobes.

Four different categories of wound are now recognized, each with its own predictable rate of infection:

1. *Clean wounds* – aseptic wounds properly prepared prior to making the incision, such as a mastectomy wound in which infection rates of between 1% and 4% can be expected.
2. *Clean-contaminated wounds* – in which either the gastrointestinal or the respiratory tract have been entered without significant spillage. Infection rate 5–15%.
3. *Contaminated wounds* – in which gross spillage from the gastrointestinal tract or an infected biliary or urinary tract has occurred. In this group in the absence of prophylactic measures infection rates of 15–25% can be expected.
4. *Grossly contaminated wounds* – dirty wounds in which the wound surfaces are directly contaminated by purulent material. In these, infection rates in excess of 25% can be expected.

CHEMOPROPHYLAXIS

With the passage of time it has become clear the chemoprophylaxis has an important part to play in the prevention of infection. In certain circumstances the indications are absolute, whilst in others, although relative, it has been clearly shown that morbidity due to infection can be greatly reduced.

Absolute indications

a. Dental extraction or manipulation in patients suffering from valvular heart disease or in whom prosthetic valves have been used, thus avoiding the dangers of subacute bacterial endocarditis or infection of the valves themselves.
b. Wounds contaminated by soil or dirty clothing in which much devitalized tissue is present, thus avoiding the danger of tetanus and gas gangrene.
c. Following splenectomy, particularly in children, to avoid the risk of pneumococcal infections.

Relative indications

It is now accepted surgical procedure to use chemoprophylaxis in all operations in which spillage from the gastrointestinal tract or an infected urinary tract may occur. In general, effective prophylaxis is only obtained if high blood and tissue levels are achieved at the time that bacterial contamination is most likely to occur. In order to achieve this aim, it is usual to administer the antibiotic of choice prior to and during the operation itself.

Over the years, many different trials have been performed to find the most effective drug and the most effective timing of administration. Drug schedules have therefore changed; for example, both Clindamycin and Lincomycin were once extensively used to prevent infection following large bowel surgery but, chiefly because of the hazards associated with pseudomembranous colitis caused by these drugs, both have now been abandoned. So far as gastrointestinal surgery was concerned, the picture was dramatically altered by the introduction of metronidazole in the late 1960's by the French pharmaceutical firm, Rhone Poulenc, who originally marketed the drug as an effective antitrichomonal agent. Its use in colorectal surgery was established in the late 1970s when a series of papers by Willis and his coworkers indicated the efficacy of metronidazole first in gynaecological surgery and later in colorectal surgery. However, as was recently pointed out by Eykyn, it is interesting to note that the discovery of this drug's remarkable activity against anaerobic organisms as opposed to protozoa was serendipitous; it arose from a letter to the Lancet in 1962 by a London dentist, who reported that a patient suffering from acute ulcerative gingivitis had apparently been cured by metronidazole given for the treatment of her vaginal trichomoniasis.

Prophylactic antimicrobial therapy in colorectal surgery

The incidence of septic complications following colorectal surgery ranges from 35 to 60%, according to reported series. It varies according to the site of the operation, being greater after left-sided than right-sided resections, and is greater still if anterior resection is required rather than a simpler sigmoid colectomy. This latter feature is due to the high rate of leakage from the lower anastomosis. In one series, in which anastomotic integrity was investigated by using water-soluble contrast media, it was found that approximately one-third of all anastomoses leaked although only in one-third of these did a faecal fistula develop. A further factor influencing the rate of sepsis in colorectal surgery is the primary disease, inflammatory bowel disease requiring resection; this is followed by a much higher rate of infection than resections performed for malignant disease.

The chief organisms responsible for sepsis following colorectal surgery are the aerobic coliforms, *Proteus* sp., *Pseudomonas aeruginosa* and the anaerobic streptococci, *Bacteroides* sp. and the *Clostridium* sp. In an effort to reduce the incidence of sepsis, and prior to the antibiotic era, surgeons attempted to diminish the faecal residue in the colon by using aperients, enemata and rectal washouts. However, although such measures reduce the bulky stools in patients not suffering from intestinal obstruction, there appears to be little if any reduction in the concentration of faecal flora. In 1941, following the introduction of the sulphonamides, first succinylsulphathiazole and later phthalylsulphathiazole were used in conjuction with mechanical methods of bowel preparation with limited success. With the coming of the antibiotic era, first neomycin and later clindomycin were used, the latter drug being introduced when it became apparent that the *Bacteroides* sp. were of great importance. When metronidazole was introduced and its importance demonstrated by Willis and coworkers it became, together with a cephalosporin, the mainline prophylactic drug, combined with improved methods of 'cleaning' the bowel of its contents. One such method – known as 'whole gut irrigation' – was described by Crapp and others in 1975. This technique consists of infusing normal saline into the gastrointestinal tract until the fluid passed per rectum is clear. A somewhat simpler alternative to this regime is to give the patient 2 litres of water to drink followed by 100 g of mannitol in a further 500 ml. The nausea induced by this treatment is controlled by giving metachlorpropamide (Maxalon) 10 mg by injection. So far as the antibiotic regime is concerned, a number of different regimes have been proposed, including;

Neomycin 1 g orally 12, 5 and 1 hour preoperatively
Metronidazole 400 mg orally, 12, 5 and 1 hour preoperatively.
Cephradine 500 mg by intramuscular injection 1 hour preoperatively.

By the use of the above methods the incidence of infected wounds and clinically important dehiscence of anastomoses can be greatly reduced.

Acute appendicitis and cholecystectomy

A large number of prospective, randomized, double-blind trials have been performed showing that the incidence of post-appendicectomy and post-cholecystectomy sepsis can be reduced by similar regimes to those described above, excluding of course the preliminary clearing of the bowel.

However, in some trials, whilst the incidence of wound infection occurring whilst the patient is still in hospital has fallen dramatically, many infections have been found to 'surface' some days later when the patient has returned home and when this is taken into account, the overall infection rate is not significantly lowered.

8 The aetiology and management of anaerobic infections

INTRODUCTION

Anaerobic infections are caused by three main groups of organisms: clostridia, bacteriodes and the anaerobic or microaerophilic streptococci.

Clostridial infections. These are responsible for three potentially lethal infections:

1. Gas and non-gas forming gangrene.
2. Tetanus.
3. Botulism.

Gas gangrene is rare. It occurs following:

a. Wounds associated with severe crushing of the tissues.
b. Occasionally, infection of above knee amputations.
c. Penetrating wounds or surgery involving the large bowel or rectum.

Tetanus is also a rare disease which could be entirely eliminated if every individual was immunized with tetanus toxoid in childhood. In many patients no overt wound is present at the time of presentation with the disease, although to acquire the infection a wound is required.

Botulism, also rare, is caused by *Clostridium botulinum* and is a particularly virulent form of food poisoning.

Bacteroidal infections. Bacteroides are Gram-negative strict anaerobes of which many varieties have now been recognized. The most pathogenic is *Bacteroides fragilis* but this forms a minority of the intestinal species of bacteroides. It causes soft tissue infections alone or in combination with *Bacteroides melaninogenicus*, *Peptostreptococcus*, or the aerobic Gram-negative bacilli.

Streptococcal infections. The anaerobic or microaerophilic streptococci frequently act synergistically with the haemolytic *Staphylococcus aureus* to produce a rare but severe form of cellulitis sometimes called Melaney's ulceration or synergistic gangrene.

CLOSTRIDIAL INFECTIONS

Gas gangrene

Bacteriology

The clostridia are saprophytes. All are spore-forming obligate anaerobes. Both vegetative and spore forms are widespread in soil, sand and faeces. They are, generally, fastidious anaerobes requiring a low redox potential to grow and to initiate conversion of the spores to vegetative, toxin-producing forms. Their presence in the bowel means that endogenous infections are possible, examples of which are puerperal sepsis following criminal abortion and gas gangrene of a thigh stump following amputation for arterial insufficiency.

The spores of the clostridia represent a highly resistant resting phase able to germinate when the surrounding conditions are propitious. The spores of *Clostridium botulinum* can withstand a temperature of 100°C for 3–5 hours, a feature which led to the abandonment of simple sterilization by boiling.

In any case of gas gangrene, several different species of organism may be found. These include two chief varieties: the saccharolytic, which include *Cl. perfringens (welchii)* which is recovered in approximately 80% of patients, *Cl. novyi (oedematiens)* and *Cl. septicum*; and the proteolytic saphrophytes, *Cl. sporogenes* and *Cl. histolyticum*.

Each organism produces a plethora of toxins all of which are important in the production of disease. For example, the lethal action of *Cl. perfringens* is proportional to the rate of production of alpha toxin, which is a necrotizing lethinase responsible for breaking down cell membranes; in addition, collagenases, hyaluronidases, proteases, lipases and a haemolysin are produced. This combination of toxins devitalizes the tissue cells and destroys the local microcirculation, thus allowing the infection to spread at an astonishing rate.

Although endogenous infection can occur, most are exogenous, the bacteria being introduced into an accidental wound in which the correct requirements are present for multiplication. The ideal environment for growth is heavy contamination of the wound with soil, severe disruption of the blood supply to the tissues and the presence of a foreign body. All investigators are agreed that whereas there is a high incidence of wound contamination there is a low incidence of actual disease. The spores and vegetative bacilli cannot initiate infection in healthy tissues, presumably because the oxygen tension is too high and they are unable to avoid destruction by phagocytosis. Various reported series have put the wound contamination rate as high as 39% and Lowbury found that 35% of burns were contaminated with *Cl. welchii* even though not a single case of gas gangrene occurred in 454 patients. In such cases, neither significant local nor systemic manifestations occur, although a brown seropurulent exudate may develop on the wound surface. This condition is not invasive because the surrounding tissues are basically healthy and the organisms are confined to the necrotic surface tissues.

Pathology

If contamination leads to active infection, the pathological process which follows is the result of the combined assault on the tissues of both the saccharolytic and proteolytic organisms, the powerful exotoxins of the former allowing the proteolytic saprophytes to develop. Either a cellulitis or the more serious myositis may develop. Either may be gas-forming or non-gas forming, the former representing the more serious form of infection.

Once established, the disease spreads because of two factors. Firstly, the organisms themselves produce enzymes which disrupt the tissue planes. Secondly, the pressure within the tissues rises because of exudation and gas formation leading to increasing ischaemia. Before putrefaction begins the muscles are brick-red and odourless, but once progressive putrefaction occurs as a result of proteolytic clostridia, the dead muscle decomposes and becomes greenish-black in colour. The gas of gas gangrene is at first odourless and is composed chiefly of hydrogen and carbon dioxide produced from muscle carbohydrate by the saccharolytic organisms. Later, when the dead tissue, now brick-red in colour, is attacked by the proteolytic organisms, the foul odour of hydrogen sulphide develops.

This local process is accompanied by severe toxaemia and progressive haemolytic anaemia due to the circulating exotoxins. Throughout the process of tissue destruction polymorphonuclear leucocytes are few in number, whilst the tissues and oedema fluid contain large numbers of organisms.

Clinical presentation

If the organisms are confined to the superficial tissues, producing a clostridial cellulitis, the incubation period between contamination and overt infection may be several days. The dissection occurs superficial to the deep fascia and may spread at an extremely rapid rate, producing discolouration of the skin as well as an increasing area of crepitus. The relative mildness of the ensuing toxaemia distinguishes the condition from a clostridial myositis.

When the infection is deeper and involves the muscles, the incubation period may be as little as six hours although more commonly it is around two days. The first symptom is often pain which is disproportionate to the degree of injury, and this is followed by increasing oedema of the affected part. In the early stages gas or crepitus may not be obvious, and it is the infrequency of the infection and the surgeon's natural unfamiliarity with the condition in civilian life which may delay diagnosis. Eventually, however, the skin becomes discoloured and vesicles appear from which there is a brown malodorous discharge. If the infection is gas-forming, crepitus is now found on palpation. At a later stage, as necrosis occurs, the skin becomes black and severe toxaemia associated with a tachycardia which is disproportionate to the degree of pyrexia develops. Jaundice due to haemolysis occurs in approximately a quarter of patients suffering from clostridial myositis, and uraemia also occurs in a quarter of patients. This latter is a serious complication, approximately 50% of the patients dying despite dialysis.

Finally septic shock develops, at which stage, near to death, the organisms may invade the blood stream and produce the classical foamy liver. The time between infection and death may be as short as 1–3 days and if there is very severe muscle damage initially the full clinical picture may develop within 6 hours.

Differential diagnosis

Diffuse clostridial myositis is most often confused with other gas-producing infections which are usually caused by mixtures of Gram-negative bacilli and Gram-positive cocci. These mixed infections are not usually as virulent as gas gangrene and respond well to incision and drainage. Crepitant cellulitis should not be confused with clostridial gangrene since it too is well treated by lesser means. Gas in the tissues is not a good differentiating point, since some species of clostridia such as *Cl. novyi* do not produce gas; non-clostridial organisms, e.g. *Escherichia coli*, often produce gas, and air may enter the tissues through a penetrating wound or from the chest.

In addition, a crepitant myositis can also be produced by anaerobic streptococci. Unlike a clostridial myositis, the clinical course is insidious and associated with marked oedema and pain. Any discharge from the wound contains large numbers of polymorphonuclear leucocytes and Gram-positive cocci, in contrast to the rods of a clostridial infection which are associated with very few leucocytes.

Other aerobic organisms may occasionally produce a crepitant lesion, including *E. coli* and *Pseudomonas aeruginosa*. These anaerobic aerogenic infections are less virulent than either the clostridial or anaerobic streptococcal lesions and only rarely involve the deeper tissues.

Diagnosis

The cornerstones of diagnosis are, firstly, the clinical history and the appearance of the wound and, secondly, bacteriological confirmation that the organisms are present. Specimens of exudate from the wound should be taken for both microscopic examination and culture under anaerobic conditions. If gas gangrene is present, a Gram stain of the exudate will show the presence of Gram-positive bacilli, although *Cl. oedematiens* may appear relatively scanty even in an active infection.

Treatment

1. Prophylaxis. It should be clearly stated that many cases of gas gangrene can be prevented if early and adequate debridement of a severe soft tissue wound is performed and, at the same time, adequate doses of parenteral benzyl penicillin are administered, giving up to 10 million units daily in divided doses intramuscularly for several days. An alternative, if the patient is capable of oral feeding, is phenoxymethyl penicillin 500 mg every four hours.

Should the patient give a history of sensitivity to this drug, a tetra-cycline should be given instead.

2. Gas gangrene antitoxin. A second line of treatment is the use of polyvalent gas gangrene antitoxin both before and after surgery, 50 000 units every six hours for 48 hours. Preliminary testing for sensitivity to horse serum is necessary since hypersensitivity reactions are not uncommon. The most commonly used antitoxin is 'mixed gas gangrene antitoxin' which is a mixture of *Cl. oedematiens, septicum* and *welchii*; the antitoxin is normally administered intravenously.

3. Hyperbaric oxygen. In 1947 a case was reported of the successful treatment of a case of spreading gas gangrene of the upper limb by the direct injection of oxygen into the affected tissues. This was followed in 1961 by a report by Brummelkamp on the dramatic arrest of the disease by exposure of the patient to oxygen at a pressure of three atmospheres. The physiological basis for this form of therapy was described in the latter part of the last century by Haldane, who showed that only 0.3 vol% of oxygen in the blood is carried in a simple solution in the plasma. When, however, the body is exposed to three atmospheres, the amount of oxygen in solution can be increased to 4 vol%. Because the partial pressure of the oxygen is also raised, the rate of diffusion of oxygen from the plasma into the tissues is increased. This form of therapy is not without its risks, as decompression sickness, joint pains, respiratory, circulatory and neurological crises can occur. The action of hyperbaric oxygen in clostridial infections is considered to be the suppression of toxin production. Once toxin production is halted, the disease cycle is broken and the spread of the disease ceases. It is claimed by those who have experience of this method of treatment that surgery can then be limited to incisions into areas of massive necrosis and that excision can be delayed until resolution of the disease, thus reducing the amount of tissue which needs to be excised.

Tetanus

The causative organism of tetanus is *Clostridium tetani*. During the 1960s, 17 people died each year from this disease but, with the increasing use of triple vaccine, diptheria, pertussis and tetanus, this figure was approximately halved by the 1980s. A complete course of toxoid consists of three spaced doses of toxoid with 6 weeks between the first and the second doses, and 6–12 months between the second and third.

Tetanus is an intoxication rather than an infection; the organism growing in the wound is not itself invasive and of itself is harmless. However, if the oxygen tension of the tissues falls or an exogenous infection is introduced together with a foreign body, tetanus spores may germinate.

Two toxins are produced by the bacillus:

1. A neurotoxin called tetanospasmin which reaches the central nervous system by passing along the motor trunks and thus interferes with inhibition of the motor neurones.
2. A haemolytic toxin known as tetanolysin.

Clinical presentation

The incubation period varies from a few days to a few weeks. Occasionally, the toxin is produced in such small amounts that it becomes fixed in the anterior horn cells of a particular segment, producing only local spasms. In more severe cases, a generalized disease occurs which is ushered in by the development of cramps and twitching of the muscles around the site of the wound followed by increased reflexes in the extremities, trismus, difficulty in swallowing, neck stiffness, headache, backache, restlessness and anxiety. When fully developed, frank generalized convulsions occur associated with opisthotonus. In the past, death was the result of apnoea during a convulsion but at the present time is more likely to be due to a respiratory complication. In general, the earlier the onset of the above clinical picture the more serious is the disease.

Diagnosis

The diagnosis is made by bacteriological examination of the material obtained from the wound, which may well have been so trivial that it passed unnoticed by the patient. The organism is described as drum-shaped, because the rod-shaped bacillus carries a terminal spore.

Prophylaxis

To prevent the development to tetanus at some future date, a child should be actively immunized using tetanus vaccine containing alum-absorbed toxoid. The primary course is normally given in the form of triple vaccine at school entry and followed by a booster dose in the teens. Even without injury, a booster dose is recommended after ten years, such treatment usually being considered to confer long lasting immunity.

Treatment of a wounded individual

In 1975, the Central Public Health Laboratory published its advice concerning the treatment of individuals suffering from wounds. They concluded that equine, bovine and other animal antitoxins were now obsolete, and that antimicrobials no longer played a primary role in the prevention of tetanus after wounding. This latter statement followed a long lasting controversy in the mid 1960s when, as an alternative to the administration of animal-derived antitoxin, many were advocating the administration of large doses of benzyl penicillin stating that this was effective in preventing the development of tetanus after wounding. The recommended treatment following injury is now determined in part by the nature of the wound and in part by the immune status of the individual. Thus patients can be divided into four categories:

Category A. Patients who have received a complete course of toxoid and a booster dose within 5 years prior to wounding. These patients require no treatment.

Category B. Patients who have received a complete course of toxoid and have received a booster dose more than 5 years, but less than 10 years prior to injury.

Treatment. One booster dose of vaccine only. The aim of the booster is to stimulate an increase in circulating antitoxin and to compensate for the possibility that patients may have responded inadequately to tetanus toxoid administered previously; this particularly concerns those patients who received plain toxoid, adsorbed toxoid only being introduced into the United Kingdom in 1963.

Category C. Patients who have received a complete course of toxoid but have not received a booster for more than 10 years.

Treatment.

1. If the wound is considered clean only a booster is required.
2. If the wound is considered dirty and a potential hazard,

human-derived tetanus (HT) antitoxin should be given
together with a booster dose of toxoid.

Human antitoxin can be obtained from HIV-negative donors via
the Blood Transfusion Service. The human-derived tetanus
antitoxin provides passive immunity; immunity requiring the
maintenance of a serum concentration of antitoxin greater than
0.01 units/ml until toxin production in the wound ceases. An intramuscular injection of 250 units of HT antitoxin will provide such a
level for approximately four weeks, and if the wound is not healed
within that time a second dose should be given. One of the great
advantages of human- as opposed to animal-derived (AT)
antitoxin is that reactions to its administration are rare; approximately 2.5% of those receiving animal-derived antitoxin developed
anaphylactic shock.

Category D. Those patients who do not know whether or not
they have been immunized in the past.

Treatment. If a clean wound has been sustained a complete
course of vaccine should be given. For all other wounds a complete course of vaccine together with 250 units of AT immunoglobulin.

The treatment of established tetanus

The treatment of established tetanus is complex but has two essential aims: (1) to reduce and neutralize the toxin which is being
produced; and (2) to control the respiratory complications of the
disease.

Antitoxin should be given in doses of between 10 000 and
50 000 units intravenously.

If mild spasms are taking place, tranquillizing drugs such as
diazpam may be sufficient to control them.

In severe cases, however, total paralysis with neuromuscular
blocking agents may be required, in which case respiration must
be maintained by means of a tracheostomy and intermittent
partial pressure ventilation. Such treatment calls for devoted
nursing and skilled anaesthesia and, depending on the severity of
the condition, may have to be maintained for many weeks. Even
when the spasms are controlled, death may still occur from
overwhelming toxaemia within the first two or three weeks of onset
of the disease.

At intervals, the relaxant is withheld to observe whether recurrent spasms develop. Obviously the absence of spasms means that the patient can be weaned from the respirator.

NON-CLOSTRIDIAL ANAEROBIC INFECTIONS

These include lesions caused by anaerobic or microaerophilic streptococci, *E. coli* and members of the bacteriodes group, notably *B. fusiformis*.

Streptococcol anaerobic infections

Lesions caused by the anaerobic streptococcus include the following.

Cancrum oris and noma vulva

These are mucocutaneous gangrenous lesions involving the mouth or vulva in which anaerobic streptococci are commonly harboured. They occur in childhood, usually associated with malnutrition and frequently preceded by an infectious illness such as measles. Both conditions produce a slow but relentless necrosis of the perioral or vulval tissues causing massive destruction of the involved tissues.

Melaney's synergistic gangrene

This condition was first described by Luckett in 1909 and in its classic form produces a gangrenous area on the abdominal wall. The lesion characteristically follows accidental or deliberate trauma to the abdomen and its contents. Frequently, tension sutures have been used to close the wound producing areas of potential tissue necrosis. The lesion starts as a small painful ulcer which slowly spreads, the ulcerated area being surrounded by a rim of gangrenous skin which is itself encircled by a purple area. Brewer and Melaney, in 1926, found that the lesion could not be produced by an injection of a haemolytic streptococcus alone, but required a mixture of streptococcus together with *Staphylococcus aureus*. The lesion has thus become known as the 'progressive synergistic gangrene of Melaney', although it has since been recognized that other organisms, such a *Proteus vulgaris* and *Staphylococcus albus*, may play a synergistic role in the condition as well.

Fournier's gangrene

First described in 1884, this lesion causes a fulminating necrosis of the scrotal skin leaving the testes exposed.

BACTEROIDES INFECTION

The third group of organisms which may become pathogenic are the bacteriodes. This group of strict anaerobes is composed of a large number of non-sporing pleomorphic organisms which may be tapered, fusiform, slender rods or branching or rounded bodies. The common members are *Bacteriodes fragilis*, *B. funduliformis*, *B. nigrescens* and *B. fusobacterium*. They are normal inhabitants of the upper respiratory tract, the vagina and the intestines, constituting more than 97% of the normal faecal flora. They inhabit not only the large bowel but also the ileum and the jejunum, a fact which was not appreciated until anaerobic cultures were made of the small bowel contents. Their association with a variety of gangrenous suppurative lesions was first recognized in 1897 by Veillon and Zubber, and they have since been isolated and described as pathogens in infections in various sites in the body. However, the importance of these organisms was fully recognized only relatively recently, because their strictly anaerobic character means that they are not identifiable on routine bacteriological examination. It has now been established that they are present in the majority of wounds which become infected following the removal of infective lesions from the abdominal cavity.

Septicaemia may occur but is rare, producing metastatic abscesses within the liver, lungs, brain or bone. Characteristically the superficial lesion produced by the bacteriodes group is foul-smelling. The pathological significance of the organism must be recognized if, despite apparently adequate antibiotic therapy, an infected lesion continues to progress. The treatment of choice is the administration of metronidazole; in adults and children over 12 years of age the dose is 400 mg three times a day.

9 Causes and treatment of shock in the surgical patient

DEFINITION

The term, 'shock' is derived from the Dutch word 'schokken' meaning to jolt suddenly. Whatever the derivation of the word it is difficult to find a definition of shock which meets with the general approval of both laboratory workers and clinicians. The clinician most commonly uses the term when referring to patients suffering from acute systemic hypotension – a condition usually, but not always, associated with pallor, weakness, sweating and a rapid thready pulse. Most laboratory workers, however, feel that this definition is too vague and that, at the very least the term, 'shock' should be qualified by the presumed cause. At the present time, most people would accept that 'shock' is a condition in which there is a persistent deficiency of bloodflow through the peripheral vascular bed, leading to inadequate perfusion of the tissues. Whatever the pathological cause of shock, there are only three significant factors at work: cardiac activity, circulating volume and the functional integrity of the peripheral vascular bed. There are three types of shock to which the Dutch word is highly appropriate: anaphylactic, neurogenic and cardiogenic shock. In each, events occur with dramatic suddenness.

ANAPHYLACTIC SHOCK

Anaphylactic shock was first described by Richet and Portier in 1902 after they had investigated the severe reactions which occurred in dogs following repeated injections of toxins derived from sea anenomes. This type of shock occurs in individuals predisposed to develop abnormal quantities of IgE antibody in response to an antigenic stimulus. It can be caused by a variety of drugs, foreign proteins and insect bites.

Typically, prior exposure to an antigen leads to the formation of significant quantities of IgE which become fixed to the basophils and mast cells. A subsequent encounter with the antigen triggers the release from these cells of a variety of substances, including histamine, SRS-A, leukotrienes, C4, D4, E4 and other factors such as heparin. In sufficient quantities, these chemicals cause vascular collapse, bronchospasm, laryngeal oedema, itching and urticaria. This form of shock is one of the many complications of penicillin and related antibiotics. The World Health Organisation estimated the frequency of anaphylactic shock after penicillin at between 0.015 and 0.04% of patients treated, with a fatality rate of between 0.0015 and 0.002%. Of those dying, approximately 70% had previously received penicillin and the remainder were suffering from fungal infections, usually of the interdigital clefts of the feet.

Treatment

This form of shock is usually treated by the injection of 0.5 – 1 ml of adrenaline intramuscularly or 0.2 ml well diluted injected intravenously and, later, by glucocorticoids.

NEUROGENIC SHOCK

The simplest and the usually most benign form of neurogenic shock is the vasovagal attack frequently caused by confrontation with an unpleasant sight or event. Two factors operate to produce the abrupt collapse of the individual: extensive vasodilatation in the splanchnic area causing a sudden reduction in the peripheral resistance, a temporary loss of venous return and a sudden fall in the blood supply to the vital centres and, in addition, vagal stimulation of the heart causing bradycardia. The mere act of falling to the ground as the individual faints, assists the haemodynamic situation and helps in recovery.

Very infrequently, a similar mechanism causes sudden death, as in pleural or obstetrical shock. The author has seen only one example of the former situation, which occurred when a patient admitted to a casualty department with fractured ribs was being treated by an injection of local anaesthetic into the chest wall.

Sudden extreme vasodilatation also occurs in patients suffering from a high transection of the cord due to a spinal fracture or following a spinal anaesthetic. In both cases, the effects are due to sympathetic paralysis causing splanchnic dilatation.

It should also be noted that a severe injury may precipitate neurogenic shock prior to the effects of hypovolaemia.

CARDIOGENIC SHOCK

The commonest causes of cardiogenic shock leading to sudden 'collapse' are acute myocardial infarction, massive pulmonary embolus and cardiac tamponade due to penetrating wounds of the chest involving the heart. Less acute causes of cardiogenic shock include low cardiac output following cardiac surgery and myocarditis.

The clinical manifestations are chiefly caused by the gross reduction of cardiac output when the systolic and diastolic pressures fall, the former usually to a greater degree than the latter. The low cardiac output leads to compensatory peripheral constriction and a cold sweaty skin. Deterioration leads to increasingly inadequate tissue perfusion and increasing metabolic acidosis.

Treatment

When the cause is sudden coronary occlusion, the outlook is dependent on the degree of damage to the myocardium. In the conscious patient, potent analgesics must be given to relieve pain, and oxygen should be administered together with drugs to improve myocardial contractility. Among the latter are the cathecholamines and digitalis glycosides.

Dopamine, which is a cathecholamine, has a powerful action on the β_1 adrenergic receptors and is given in a dose of between 1–30 µg/kg per minute.

Digoxin is administered in a dose of 0.5 mg in saline over 30 minutes followed by a further 0.5 mg over two hours, after which a maintenance dose is required.

If the cardiac output remains inadequate but the peripheral blood pressure remains high, i.e. above 90 mmHg (12.0 kPa) a reduction in the ventricular afterload may assist the patient and this can be achieved by the use of an α-adrenergic antagonist such as phentolamine, 0.1–0.2 µg/minute or salbutamol which is a β_2 agonist, 0.5–1.6 µg/minute.

Cardiac massage and artificial respiration. Should cardiac arrest occur, there is an abrupt loss of consciousness accompanied by gasping respiration and an associated absence of cardiac and major peripheral pulses. As time progresses, and within three or four minutes the cerebrum is damaged beyond repair, the pupils dilate and the skin becomes ashen grey. Because of the need to restore the cerebral blood flow it is imperative that cardiac massage is commenced immediately.

External massage in modern times was first described by Koenig in 1883 and is acceptable in all the categories noted above except in cases of tamponade. The technique is as follows. A board or tray is placed under the thorax and a compression force is delivered to the chest by means of the heel of the hand, the hand being hyper-extended at the wrist and the arm extended at the elbow, the left hand normally lying over the right in a right-handed individual. The thrust is delivered not by movements of the arm and forearm but by the bodyweight. The aim is to compress the heart between the sternum in front and the spine behind. In order to achieve this, compression should be applied at the junction of the upper two-thirds of the sternum with the lower one-third. If compression is applied too vigorously, costochondral disclocations may follow, ribs may be broken, the stomach may be ruptured or damage to the liver may occur.

As the seconds pass the need to commence artificial respiration becomes more urgent. Three methods are possible but of course may not be available: expired air resuscitation, mouth to mouth or mouth to nose; bag/valve/mask system; respiration through a cuffed endotracheal tube.

If cardiac massage and artificial respiration are successful, the brain will at least be protected from total anoxia, and in the patient who was previously conscious some indication of success should be obtained from evidence of increasing cerebral activity. The enlarged pupils should begin to diminish in size, the eyelash reflex should return, muscle tone should improve and spontaneous respiratory efforts should return.

HYPOVOLAEMIC SHOCK

Hypovolaemic shock may be due to loss of electrolytes and fluid, loss of plasma or loss of whole blood. At the present time, haemorrhage is the commonest cause of hypovolaemic shock seen by the surgeon. Fluid and electrolyte imbalance is now relatively easily prevented and a number of measures in industry have greatly reduced the number of major burns which were in the past the commonest cause of plasma loss.

Haemorrhagic shock

The response to excessive blood loss depends on the volume and the rapidity with which it occurs.

When the loss is moderate, as for example the sudden withdrawal of some 500 ml as occurs in a blood donor, little reaction occurs in the healthy individual. This is because the venous reservoirs, the large veins, the cutaneous venous plexus, spleen, liver and intestines which contain 70% of the total blood volume contract, with the result that little if any physiological disturbance occurs. Such a loss may, however, be important in an ageing atherosclerotic individual or in a patient on antihypotensive drugs which prevent the necessary compensatory vasoconstriction occurring.

In the course of a few hours, fluids and electrolytes are drawn from the interstitial compartment producing a degree of haemodilution which can be measured by estimating either the haematocrit or the haemoglobin. The lost serum protein is replaced within hours, as also is the interstitial water due to a reduced excretion of water and salt caused by an increased secretion of ADH. When the loss increases to 1000 ml, the systolic blood pressure may fall to 90 mm Hg and the patient may exhibit, albeit temporarily, the classic signs of 'shock'; i.e. he appears anxious with a cold clammy skin and a thready pulse and observation reveals a fall in urine output. However, so long as there is no further loss, even if no treatment is given, the blood pressure returns to normal within a few hours.

If even greater losses occur, the blood pressure may remain low for some 24–48 hours during which time the adverse effects of 'shock' may develop. In this situation not only has the venous side of the circulation contracted and the heart rate and myocardial contractility increased, but in addition the systemic vascular resistance has also increased as a result of arteriolar vasoconstriction in the skin, skeletal muscles, kidneys and splanchnic area.

The body's initial response to massive blood loss is thus remarkably effective. Bloodflow to the heart and brain is maintained whilst it is reduced in regions which are more tolerant of ischaemia. However, this response cannot be maintained indefinitely and adverse changes begin to occur in due course both at the microcirculatory level and in the cells themselves. If the condition is not rectified, these changes result in the failure of organ function.

Different tissues vary in their ability to withstand hypoxia caused by derangement of the circulation and loss of the oxygen-carrying capacity of the blood attendant on the loss of red cells. For example, whereas the liver is relatively tolerant, the astrocytes of the central nervous system are highly susceptible to hypoxia. At some point, therefore, shock which is reversible becomes irreversible, and whereas even massive haemorrhage approaching 50% or more of the total blood volume may be attended by a favourable outcome if treated immediately or soon after it occurs, in time no treatment appears to be effective and death follows.

One of the first effects brought about by the failure of tissue perfusion with the associated tissue anoxia is a change in cellular metabolism from aerobic to anaerobic. Since anaerobic metabolism is less effective than aerobic, the complete breakdown of foodstuffs to carbon dioxide and water does not occur. Both lactate and adenosine triphosphate become the end products, the latter yielding abundant H ions when it is hydrolysed so that intracellular acidosis develops. In addition, changes in cell volume and in the cell membranes occurs allowing NaCl and water to leak from the extracellular compartment into the cells. Lysosomal enzymes leak into the circulation and act on precursors present in the circulation to form kinins which cause arteriolar dilatation and relaxation of the precapillary sphincters, whilst the postcapillary sphincters maintain their tone. These effects run counter to the vasoconstriction which occurred at first and, in combination with the increase in capillary permeability, promote increasing fluid loss from the circulation.

So far as organ function is concerned a variety of changes, all harmful to the whole, occur:

1. Mucosal breakdown leads to increasing permeability of the gastrointestinal tract to bacteria and their toxins and, in the stomach, mucosal ulceration causes stress ulcers to appear which further compound the problem.
2. Failure of the hepatic reticuloendothelial system leads to an inability to clear absorbed endotoxins from the circulation and allows bacteria to gain entrance into the systemic circulation.
3. Afferent arteriolar constriction in the kidney brought about by angiotensin, catecholamines and prostaglandins if persistent, leads to acute renal failure.
4. The associated tachycardia, rising end diastolic pressure and

falling arterial diastolic pressure, together with an as yet unidentified cardiogenic factor, jeopardizes myocardial function leading to heart failure.
5. Interstitial oedema, increasing arteriovenous shunting and loss or changes in surfactant in the lungs leads to the adult respiratory distress syndrome (ARDS), causing increasing hypoxia.

The point at which the prognosis becomes doubtful is reached when the acidotic state becomes extracellular and therefore readily measurable. Indeed, some investigators claim that a blood lactate above 4 mosmol/l is the dividing line; above this level the mortality can be expected to be high.

Treatment

The most appropriate treatment of haemorrhagic shock is the replacement of the deficit by blood, thus in physiological terms optimizing the ventricular preload. However, since blood is not instantaneously available, the first line of treatment after first taking a sample of blood for grouping and cross-matching is to give what can only be a temporary boost to the intravascular compartment by the intravenous administration of 1–2 litres of a balanced salt solution. This is appropriate 'first aid' treatment for all patients except those who have suffered a major chest injury accompanied by a pulmonary contusion or who have a previous history of cardiac disease associated with pulmonary oedema, for in either case the administration of such a fluid might well precipitate or exacerbate pre-existing pulmonary oedema.

A more appropriate treatment in such patients is the administration of plasma or a plasma expander. These include the dextrans – either Dextran 40 or 110, both of which are obtained from the fermentation of *Leuconostoc mesenteroides*. Approximately 60% of an infusion of Dextran 40 is excreted in the urine within six hours, and 70% within 24 hours; whereas some Dextran 110 is retained in the circulation for 2–3 days even though some 40% is excreted within 24 hours.

An alternative to the use of dextrans is the use of Polygeline Haemocell® (Hoechst) which is a polymer of molecular weight 35 000, prepared by cross-linking polypeptides derived from denatured gelatin with a di-isocyanate to form urea bridges.

When correctly cross-matched blood is available it should be given, the problem being how much. If persistent shock is present, something of the order of 1500 ml of blood must have been lost but blood loss may be well in excess of this in major trauma. Simple clinical observation together with repeated measurement of the blood pressure may help, as indeed may measurement of the urine output; a urine output of less than one-half the normal minimum volume of 1 ml/kg bodyweight per hour indicating in the acute state that the patient remains undertransfused.

Monitoring the severely shocked patient

In a patient in whom massive trauma has occurred – e.g. a road traffic victim suffering from multiple fractures and internal bleeding and in whom prolonged hypotension is present – careful monitoring of the cardiopulmonary systems are required. The measures to achieve this include:

a.   Central Venous Pressure (CVP).
b.   Pulmonary Artery Wedge Pressure (PAWP).
c.   Electrocardiography.
d.   Temperature.
e.   Blood gases.

   a. Central venous pressure. Some indication of whether volume replacement is adequate, sufficient or if overtransfusion has occurred may be gained from measuring the CVP. In precise terms, the CVP is the venous pressure in the right atrium and, assuming the tricuspid valve is functioning normally, the CVP is equal to the end-diastolic pressure in the right ventricle and is a measure of the preload to this chamber.

   To measure the CVP, a cannula is placed in the right atrium. The precise position of the cannula can be established either by screening, if it is radio-opaque, or by continuously recording the ECG using the cannula as one of the leads. As the cannula enters the atrium, the P waves become biphasic. The cannula can be inserted via the median cubital vein or the subclavian. The ideal place for the tip of the cannula is at the lower border of the superior vena cava or in the upper third of the atrium itself. Once it has been inserted, the simplest way of measuring the central venous pressure is to use a manometer containing isotonic saline set against a centimetre rule. A reference point is then chosen; in the United Kingdom this is usually the manubriosternal joint. In a patient reclining in bed supported by five or six pillows, the normal pressure measurement from this reference point is between 5 and 10 cm of water.

Since this is an invasive technique, occasional complications are inevitable. Either route of entry can become infected if not properly cared for. Catheter embolus and, sometimes, cardiac tamponade due to perforation of the right atrium have both been described. If a subclavian puncture is used, the following complications may also occasionally occur; pneumothorax, haemothorax, hydrothorax, air embolus, subcutaneous emphysema, arteriovenous fistula and brachial palsy.

Assuming that cardiac function is normal – which of course, is not necessarily so in the severely shocked patient – the CVP roughly corresponds to the blood volume. Thus, a high pressure of, say, 20 cm of water indicates plethora and the possibility of pulmonary oedema, whilst a low pressure indicates hypovolaemia. However, if cardiac function is abnormal, either through natural disease or as part of the shock syndrome, the CVP will rise above the normally accepted level of about 10 cm of water even though the patient remains undertransfused. This elevation is caused by defective function of the right side of the heart which finds itself unable to pump more blood through the pulmonary bed.

b. Pulmonary artery wedge pressure. When the right side of the heart is functioning abnormally, it is highly probable that the left side of the heart is equally affected. It has therefore become customary in intensive care units to measure the pulmonary artery wedge pressure (PAWP) to ascertain whether the left ventricle is also malfunctioning. This is done by the use of a Swan–Ganz catheter, first described in 1970. The catheter has a balloon near its tip and is introduced via the same routes as a central venous line. Once the catheter tip has reached a large intrathoracic vein, the balloon is inflated and the catheter then slowly advanced, the bloodflow carrying it through the right atrium and right ventricle onwards into a small branch of the pulmonary artery where it becomes wedged. The position of the catheter is monitored throughout its passage by pressure changes and the different wave forms which occur.

In a normal individual, the PAWP at the end of respiration and at the level of the mid-axillary line measures 6–12 mm Hg (0.8–1.6 kPa). The complications associated with the passage of a Swan–Ganz catheter are those already described for a central venous line but, in addition, arrhythmias may occur as the catheter passes through the right ventricle and, occasionally, the catheter becomes knotted in the eddying currents which it encounters.

Value of PAWP measurement. Whereas measurement of the central venous pressure gives information which can be related to the function of the right side of the heart, the PAWP gives a direct measure of left ventricular filling pressure and left ventricular function. Furthermore, it can be used to measure the blood volume and the PO_2 of mixed venous blood. It is, therefore, particularly valuable in managing patients in whom exact knowledge of left ventricular activity is required. For example, if a high central venous pressure is found in the presence of a low cardiac output it would be appropriate to think in terms of pump failure. However, if the PAWP is measured and is found to be low, the clinical condition may be one of simple hypovolaemia which can be readily corrected. When left-sided failure is not due to low preload, the PAWP will be found to be high.

c. Electrocardiography. In addition to direct measurement of cardiac function by the methods described above, an ECG is used to provide information about the heart rate and rhythm.

d. Temperature. A simple non-invasive method of assessing cardiac output and peripheral perfusion is to measure the difference between the peripheral and core temperatures. The former is measured by a sensor attached to the big toe, and the latter by a probe placed in either the rectum or the oesophagus. When the cardiac output is low and perfusion poor, the difference between the two measurements may even exceed 10°C, the difference declining as normal perfusion is restored.

e. Blood gases.

Oxygen

If measurement of the PO_2 – which should be maintained at between 70 and 100 mmHg (9.3–13.3 kPa) indicates that this is falling, oxygen should be given by face mask, nasal catheter or mechanical ventilation.

Inotropic agents

Should hypoperfusion persist after volume expansion and an increase in cardiac filling pressure, medication designed to improve myocardial contractility and hence cardiac output becomes important. This is achieved chiefly by the use of inotropic agents, such as noradrenaline and two more recently introduced inotropic drugs, dopamine and dobutamine.

Noradrenaline. This drug will increase cardiac output, but if the systolic pressure is in excess of 70–80 mmHg its action is inconsistent. Furthermore, it produces excessive vasoconstriction thus decreasing tissue perfusion still further.

Dopamine. The action of dopamine differs from that of noradrenaline and isoprenaline in that it has a renal vasodilating effect, produced apparently by activation of non-adrenergic receptor mechanisms. If dopamine is given intravenously and the systolic pressure rises to 80–100 mmHg, it will induce a diuresis.

Dobutamine. This drug acts directly on β_1-adrenergic receptors and, to a much lesser extent, on β_2- and α-adrenergic receptors. It is reported to have a more pronounced inotropic action on the heart than does isoprenaline or noradrenaline, with a negligible effect on the heart rate or on myocardial irritability.

Noradrenaline, dopamine and dobutamine all have a short half-life and must be given by continous intravenous transfusion for a sustained effect. The administration of all catecholamines should also cease as soon as possible.

Complications of blood transfusion

Blood transfusion itself is not without problems. These include:

1. *Circulatory overload* leading to pulmonary oedema.
2. *Air embolus* due to faulty transfusion technique. This produces a frothy airlock in the right ventricle and pulmonary artery. As a result, the blood pressure falls, the pulse becomes rapid and thready and a millwheel murmur can be heard over the praecordium.
3. *Transient pyrexia* due to the presence of leucocyte antibodies.
4. *Transmission of disease.*
   a. Hepatitis. The transmission of hepatitis A and B has been almost eliminated by the adequate screening of donors. However, non-A, non-B hepatitis may occur due to the transfusion of blood contaminated by cytomegalic inclusion virus, the herpes virus, the Epstein Barr virus and yellow fever.

b. AIDS. Screening of donors should eliminate this possible complication.

c. Malaria. The malarial parasite is able to survive for days or weeks in blood stored at 4°C. The only positive way to prevent transmission is to avoid using blood donors who have lived in endemic areas or to screen such individuals carefully.

5. *Incompatible blood transfusion.* This can be due to a variety of causes including:

a. The administration of cells to a recipient whose plasma contains iso-antibodies capable of damaging them. This is most commonly due to an error either of identification or of labelling.

b. The donor blood itself contains sufficient antibodies to haemolyse recipient cells.

c. Red cells of reduced viability are transfused. This is usually due to poor storage conditions or the use of outdated blood. Despite substrates and cooling to slow metabolism, a progressive slow glycolysis results in lactate accumulation and, because mature red cells do not have a Krebs Cycle to remove pyruvate and prevent lactate accumulation, a slow but inevitable rise in lactate occurs leading to a lowering of the pH and the eventual loss of red cell viability. The storage life of CPDA red cells stored at between 1 and 6°C is 35 days. A deficiency of platelets is evident within 24 hours and factors V and VIII also have a limited lifespan.

Any of these situations leads to haemolysis. This may be intravascular, if brought about by antibodies which are haemolytic in vitro, or extravascular, when caused by antibodies that cannot cause haemolysis in vitro. The presence of intravascular haemolysis is confirmed by finding that the plasma is discoloured by haemoglobin, and the presence of haemoglobinuria. When extravascular haemolysis occurs, the cells are taken up by the reticuloendothelial system, haemoglobinaemia does not occur, but a transient increase in serum bilirubin occurs for some 12–36 hours.

In the unconscious patient, the only signs of a mismatched transfusion may be the development of inexplicable hypotension and generalized oozing.

In the conscious patient, an incompatible transfusion usually gives rise to symptoms within 20 minutes. A feeling of warmth may spread up the limb through which the transfusion is being administered, to be followed by chills, fever, backache and hypotension. Tightness of the chest may give rise to pain; the cause of this is doubtful but may be due to agglutinates blocking the pulmonary arteries or the liberation of histamine-like substances constricting the bronchial vessels and bronchioles. About 75 ml of blood are sufficient to produce a reaction, and a transfusion of some 200 ml may be fatal. Should the patient survive a sublethal imcompatible transfusion, renal failure or disseminated intravascular coagulation may follow. Much depends on the condition of the kidneys prior to the assault and on the presence or absence of gross physiological disturbance of the renal circulation at the time of transfusion. Thus, the presence of hypovolaemic shock may result in the deposition of haemoglobin or its degradation products. Although haemoglobin itself may block the renal tubules, the major factor causing renal damage appears to be the stroma of the damaged red cells. An antigen/antibody reaction occurs which produces renal ischaemia, later to be followed by renal failure.

The initial treatment of a mismatched blood transfusion should be the administration of 20 g of mannitol in a 20% solution over 10 minutes, and not more than 80 g over the first 24 hours.

6. *Hypothermia*. Clinically significant lowering of the body temperature will occur if several units of blood which is normally stored at 4°C are given without prior warming. Storage at this temperature slows the metabolism.

7. *Citrate intoxication*. Stored blood contains 2.63 g citrate per unit of blood. This is part of the anticoagulant preservative which also contains phosphate, dextrose and adenine. Since citrate binds to calcium, which is essential for the coagulation cascade, it serves as an anticoagulant. In theory, too much citrate could therefore lower the calcium to such a degree that hypocalcaemia could occur. However, in practice this complication is seldom seen except in patients with severe liver dysfunction who cannot metabolise citrate.

In a previously healthy adult, major clinical problems are associated only with massive transfusion of some 7–10 units within a 24 hour period, and are chiefly due to thrombocytopenia and hypothermia. The blood should therefore be warmed and a prophylactic platelet transfusion should be given if more than 10 units of packed cells have been administered.

Treatment of hypovolaemic shock due to burns

When burning or scalding occurs, a protein-rich exudate escapes from the affected surface and this continues, although at an ever diminishing rate, over the first 48 hours. If the affected area exceeds 10% of the body surface area in a child, or 18% in an adult, hypovolaemic shock will occur if no resuscitatory measures are taken. The area burnt can be estimated by the rule of nine, first devised by Polaski and Tennison but often referred to as the Wallace Rule. From the standpoint of immediate resuscitation the depth of the burn can be ignored, since the volume of plasma lost is determined by the area affected rather than the depth. However in whole thickness, as opposed to partial thickness burns, red cell loss does occur due to a number of causes, and it has been estimated that 20% of the red cell volume is lost in a burn involving 50% of the total surface area of the body. It is therefore mandatory to administer whole blood at some point in the treatment of extensive whole thickness burns.

In addition to the escape of protein-rich exudate, the loss of the covering skin also leads to loss of water from the burn by-evaporation. Normally, the water lost by evaporation in a temporate climate is approximately equal to 15 ml/m^2 per hour, but in a severe burn the loss rises perhaps to as much as 200 ml/m^2 per hour. This evaporative loss is accompanied by a corresponding heat loss, 1 g of water evaporated from the body representing a loss of 0.575 kcal. Since the evaporated water is virtually sodium-free, an underestimation of the rate of loss may rapidly lead to the development of hypertonic dehydration due to hypernatraemia.

Other indications, in addition to the extent of the area burnt, that resuscitation is required are:

1. A deterioration of the general condition of the patient.
2. A rising pulse rate.
3. A falling blood pressure.
4. A diminishing urine output.

Types of fluid used for replacement

a. Saline in Ringer lactate. Interest in the use of saline in the treatment of burns requiring resuscitation was largely stimulated by the high cost of plasma. Some 30 years ago, it was shown that normal saline could be used almost as satisfactorily as plasma in adults, but was associated with a higher mortality in childhood.

The thinking behind the use of crystalloid is (1) that filling the extracellular space with isotonic saline increases the tissue pressure, so preventing leakage from the damaged capillaries, and (2) that sodium loss is the chief cause of burn shock. Practically, an advantage of Ringer lactate over normal saline is that the acidosis associated with the infusion of excessive chloride does not occur.

In the United Kingdom, the Birmingham Burns Unit tested the efficacy of this method of resuscitation in both children and adults and found that it was only satisfactory when the patient was closely supervised in order that a change to plasma or human purified protein fraction (HPPF) could, if necessary, be made.

b. Dried plasma. This is obtained from the supernatant fluid which is separated by centrifuging whole blood. Such plasma is supplied as a deep cream-coloured powder or friable agglomerate which dissolves completely in water in 10 minutes. The solution is yellow and contains not less than 4.5% w/v of protein.

c. Dried human purified protein fraction (HPPF). This consists mainly of albumin with a small proportion of globulins. It is administered as a 5% solution.

Both dried plasma and HPPF are heat sterilised at 60 degrees centigrade for several hours and are thus rendered free of viruses. Neither contain clotting factors.

d. Human albumin solution. This is a clear, moderately viscous, almost odourless, brownish liquid containing 4.5% albumin wt/v and 147 mmol sodium per litre. It is also available in higher concentrations when the advantage is that the intravascular oncotic pressure can be raised without giving too great a volume.

Calculation of the volume requirement

The volume of human albumin solution – now one of the most commonly used replacement fluids – can be calculated from one of many formulae.

One of the simplest rule-of-thumb methods is to give 100 ml of albumin solution for every point which the haematocrit has risen.

The author has found that the formula proposed by Muir and Barclay is satisfactory, since it recognizes that the rate of loss of plasma is greatest in the first 12 hours after burning and diminishes over the next 24 hours. This total period is subdivided into 6 periods of 4, 4, 4, 6, 6 and 12 hours.

The first step is to work out the area of the body burnt from the rule of nine, after which this figure is applied to the following formula:

$$\frac{\% \text{ area of body burnt} \times \text{weight in kg}}{2}$$

The above formula gives the volume required during each of the above intervals.

The first aliquot must be transfused within the first four hours and, even if the transfusion does not begin until, say, three hours after burning, the calculated total volume required should be given in the remaining hour.

In addition to the albumin, 100 ml of water hourly should be given by mouth to an adult if the patient does not find it nauseating, or intravenously if oral feeding is impossible.

If Ringer lactate is used, greater quantities of fluid are required. The Baxter and Shires formula, of 4 ml/kg per 1% area burnt, is used administering one-half the total volume in the first 8 hours.

When the burn is greater than 20% of the total body surface area, blood is necessary in addition to albumin. The amount required is equal to 1% of the patient's estimated blood volume for each 1% of the burnt area, the approximate blood volume being calculated from the following simple formula:

$$\text{Blood volume} = \text{weight in kg} \times 75.$$

After the theorectical requirements have been calculated, a number of other factors should be considered. Note should be taken: that young children and elderly adults will not tolerate excessive quantities of fluid; that patients with pre-existing cardiovascular or renal disease should be treated with caution; and that in flash burns, in which respiratory tract irritation may be present, pulmonary oedema is commonplace. Furthermore, extensive burns are often followed by paralytic ileus, and in these patients fluids should not be given by mouth until bowel sounds return (see also Ch. 18).

SEPTIC SHOCK

Septic shock may be caused by both Gram-positive organisms, such as the staphylococci, streptococci and clostridia, and by a large number of Gram-negative organisms, including escherichia, proteus, salmonella and the anaerobic bacteriodes sp.

The chief difference between these two groups of bacteria lies in the structure and the nature of the bacterial wall. In Gram-positive organisms, the wall is relatively simple and the basic structure upon which its strength depends is composed of a mucopeptide comprising N-acetylglucosamine and N-acetyl muramic acid molecules linked alternatively in a chain. Other components such as muramic acid and glycine are also present. In Gram-negative organisms, the bacterial wall is a more complex structure made up of lipid, polysaccharide, protein and lipopolysaccharide. Whereas the toxins from Gram-positive organisms are contained within the cytoplasm and are secreted by actively dividing bacteria, the toxin of the Gram-negative organisms is the lipopolysaccheride component of the wall of the organism which is liberated only when the bacillus dies. The chief differentiating features between an exotoxin and an endotoxin are that the latter are:

1. An integral part of the outer layer of the bacterial cell.
2. Heat stable.
3. Less specific in their cytotoxic effects than are exotoxins.
4. Not convertible to toxoids.
5. Not rendered non-toxic when combined with the homolgous antibody.

Whilst sepsis in a previously healthy individual is normally readily contained, this is not necessarily the case in an individual whose host response has been altered by surgery, trauma, acute illness or pre-existing chronic disease.

Symptoms and signs

The classic symptoms of septic shock include mental confusion associated with a high fever, although in some cases hypothermia develops. Commonly, the patient develops hyperventilation which results in hypercapnia.

The chief initial sign is hypotension but if the condition persists evidence of multiple organ failure will be found, including tubular necrosis of the kidney leading to oliguria, disseminated intravascular coagulation and the adult respiratory distress syndrome.

Pathophysiology

A variety of agents have been incriminated as the causative agents of septic shock including:

1. Endogenous vasodilators such as histamine and prostacyclin.
2. Vasoconstrictor agents such as vasopressin, thromboxane, the catecholamines and angiotensin.
3. Macrophage-derived monokines concerned with the regulation of temperature, metabolism and immunological systems.
4. Activated complement components.
5. Free radicals.
6. Proteases.
7. As yet unidentified myocardial and vascular depressants.

The usual circulatory response to sepsis is vasodilatation, producing an increase in the vascular capacity with a corresponding reduction of the ventricular afterload and a corresponding increase in cardiac output. However, this response may be blunted or even eliminated if hypovolaemia or myocardial dysfunction is present due to pre-existing or intercurrent disease.

It is usually considered that warm hypotension is a feature of Gram-positive sepsis, whereas cold hypotension with peripheral shutdown indicates a Gram-negative septicaemia caused by the liberation of the lipopolysaccharide. The latter can be detected by the limulus test, in which the protein of the white cells of the horse shoe crab, *Limulus polyphemus*, is coagulated into a gel by even minute amounts of the toxic material.

Gram-negative endotoxaemia occurs whenever Gram-negative organisms disintegrate within the bloodstream or, alternatively, endotoxin is absorbed from the gastrointestinal tract. Jacob Fine of Boston postulated that the end-stage in severe hypovolaemic shock was reached when the mucosal resistance of the intestinal wall allowed endotoxin from the resident gastrointestinal bacteria to gain entrance into the bloodstream. Normally in an experimental animal such as the rabbit, sublethal doses of endotoxin are adequately dealt with by the cells of the mononuclear phagocyte system. If a lethal dose is given, death ensues from breakdown of the microvascular circulation directly attributed to the action of the endotoxin. In such an animal, it is possible to enhance the activity of these cells by repeated sublethal injections, with the result that the animal becomes resistant not only to a supralethal dose of endotoxin but also to prolonged haemorrhagic shock of such severity that the animal would normally die.

In the human, as the shock state associated with sepsis continues, proteolysis rapidly leads to profound muscle wasting and weakness. It has been shown that 30% of the energy requirements may be provided by amino acids in end stage sepsis, and that the hypercatabolic septic response may persist for a variable period despite control of the primary infection.

Diagnosis

Repeated blood cultures may be required to identify the causative organism and its sensitivity. All efforts should be made to identify local collections of pus.

Treatment

1. Antibiotics should be started immediately the condition is diagnosed and prior to confirmation of sensitivity; a combination of metronidazole and an aminoglycoside is normally advised. If this combination proves unsuitable it is changed when the sensitivity is known.

2. When a source of infection can be identified which is amenable to surgical treatment, it should be dealt with at the earliest possible moment. For example, radical improvement may occur following total colectomy in patients suffering from severe acute ulcerative colitis accompanied by toxic dilatation of the colon, and in patients suffering from faecal peritonitis as a result of perforation of the colon in whom lavage and drainage are performed.

3. H_2 antagonists should be administered in an attempt to avoid stress ulceration of the gastroduodenal mucosa.

4. Corticosteroids, e.g. dexamethasone 1.5 mg/kg, may be useful if given within 4 hours of the onset of hypotension; this dose can be repeated after a further 4 hours on the hypothesis that it might protect the microcirculation by stabilizing cell membranes. No further steroid should be given, since repeated doses cause depression of the mononuclear phagocytes.

5. Any volume defect should be replaced.

6. Cardiopulmonary function should be carefully monitored and the cardiac index maintained at greater than normal levels by the use of inotropic agents; this is because of the increased metabolic requirements in septic shock.

7. Metabolic acidosis should be corrected by the administration of bicarbonate solutions.

10 Fluid and electrolyte imbalance

INTRODUCTION

Approximately 58% of the total bodyweight is water. This large volume is divided between two compartments: the intracellular water (ICF), which accounts for some 35% of the bodyweight; and the extracellular water (ECF) which accounts for the remainder. The latter can be further subdivided into the interstitial water, accounting for some 16%, and the intravascular or plasma water, accounting for 4%, excluding the red cell component which for haemodynamic purposes behaves as a fluid. In terms of volume there are, therefore, approximately 24 litres of intracellular water, 15 litres of interstitial water and 2.8 litres of intravascular or plasma water. The three compartments are separated from one other by membranes, each having a different permeability which allows the various compartments to contain different solutes.

The chief solutes of the intravascular fluid, which are the main factor determining its tonicity, are sodium and its corresponding anions, chloride and bicarbonate, together with crystalloids such as urea and proteins. The total tonicity of the plasma is some 300 mosmols, approximately 280 mosmols being attributable to the electrolytes and about one-half of this (140 mosmol/l) to sodium; the anions combined with sodium contribute the other half. The crystalloids, sugar, urea and creatinine, account for only about 10–20 mosmol, and protein, which is so important in containing fluid within the vascular tree, accounts for only about 2 mosmols.

Tonicity is chiefly regulated by varying levels of the antidiuretic hormone (ADH), which is controlled via the hypothalamus. The administration or intake of excessive water without salt results in a reduced secretion of ADH and hence elimination of the excess water. A normal individual can void up to 20 litres per day with an osmolarity of 40 (specific gravity 1.004). Conversely, if the solute concentration rises, hypothalamic receptors stimulate the release of ADH causing an increase in the reabsorption of water by the distal convoluted tubules of the kidney. Thus, a normal individual may excrete as little as 500 ml of urine daily with an osmolarity of 1200 (specific gravity 1.040), although it has been shown that even in the absence of ADH the kidney can still conserve water by excreting a hypertonic urine.

In addition to ADH, the secretion of aldosterone also plays a significant role in the regulation of ECF volume. Aldosterone promotes the retention of sodium and the excretion of potassium by the kidney, and also stimulates sodium reabsorption from the sweat and succus entericus. The major stimuli to aldosterone secretion are a decrease in the sodium concentration or an increase in potassium concentration in the ECF; either or both of these abnormalities usually being associated with a shrinkage of the ECF volume. As sodium retention follows the release of the hormone, the blood volume increases and the blood pressure tends to rise. These effects stimulate the volume receptors of the great veins and the right auricle which in turn reflexly inhibit the release of antidiuretic hormone. In general terms, osmolarity takes precedence over volume; a 1% change in the former produces ADH secretion whereas a 6% change in the volume of the ECF can be tolerated without any change in the mass of sodium excreted.

The interstitial fluid – which is identical with plasma except for its protein and cellular elements – is separated from the intravascular space by the capillary membrane, which is permeable to water and to all the solutes in plasma except for the protein and red cells.

The amount of fluid on one side of the membrane or the other is determined by two factors: the hydrostatic pressure on either side of the membrane, and the oncotic pressure exerted by the plasma proteins in the intravascular fluid.

The intracellular water has an entirely different solute composition to that of the ECF. The most abundant cations are potassium and magnesium. These provide the majority of the osmolality of the ICF and are attached to the large macromolecules and the anions, sulphate and phosphate. When the cell membranes are normal (as opposed to abnormal, e.g. in the so-called 'sick cell syndrome') sodium with its anion chloride is not allowed into the cell and, conversely, potassium and phosphate are retained within the cell. The cell membrane is, however, permeable to water, allowing pure water to cross freely following an osmotic gradient. Thus, should the intracellular fluid alter in tonicity, either cellular water will be drawn out of the cell, or more water will enter the cell in order to equilibrate the tonicity of the fluids on either side of the boundary. A minority of cells can, however, specifically inhibit larger shifts in their water content, by varying the number of intracellular particles. This is especially advantageous in the brain, where a large increase in cellular water would compromise the blood flow by compression or, conversely, a decrease leading to shrinkage of the brain could cause vascular connections with the calvarium to rupture leading to intracranial haemorrhage.

Under normal circumstances, the structure and volume of the ICF and ECF compartments are ultimately controlled by the kidney and, to a lesser extent, by the lungs and skin, the two latter accounting for the so-called 'insensible loss'. Normally, the respiratory loss is about 600 ml of pure water per day, and the evaporation through the skin, some 400 ml. Whilst these volumes can be increased, as in fever, they cannot be decreased; in contrast, the renal excretion of water and electrolytes can be adjusted throughout a wide range.

Normally, the daily fluid intake is between 2 and 3 litres, and on a normal dietary regime, 800 mosmol of solute have to be excreted daily. Since a healthy kidney can concentrate urine to 1200 mosmols/1, less than one litre of urine needs to be excreted daily to deal with the solute load. In the absence of a normal dietary intake, a urine output of 500 ml is adequate to deal with the solute load.

In general, the fluid and electrolye intake of a normal adult during the short postoperative period, during which no fluid is taken orally, should be approximately: water, 1500ml; sodium and chloride, $50-75$ mmol/m^2; potassium, 40 mmol. Other vital solutes need not be considered in the short term since adequate stores are available. Although there is an adequate store of potassium, since this is chiefly intracellular, it is not readily available. Children need proportionately more potassium than adults because they are growing. Reasonable values in the short term would therefore be: water, 1500 ml; sodium, $50-75$ mmol; and potassium 50 mmol/m^2 per day.

Causes of fluid and electrolyte disturbance

The commonest cause of fluid and electrolyte disturbance seen by the surgeon is the loss of gastrointestinal secretions. These losses may result from natural causes or as a consequence of surgical procedures. Natural diseases associated with abnormal losses are those which produce prolonged vomiting or diarrhoea. Vomiting is usually due to pyloric stenosis or high small bowel obstruction from whatever cause. Diarrhoea may be the result of: infection, as in gastro-jejuno-colic fistulae, pseudomembranous enterocolitis, Crohn's disease and ulcerative colitis; the excessive secretion of acid, as in the Zollinger–Ellison syndrome; or caused by tumours of the lower bowel, as in patients suffering from extensive villous tumours of the rectum, from which large volumes of fluid and potassium may be lost.

Certain operations, such as ileostomy, are automatically followed by temporary and excessive losses of fluid and sodium. Following the commencement of ileostomy function, the volume of fluid discharged from the stoma may reach 1.5 litres between the third and fifth days, but by the end of the first post-operative week, if all has gone well, the volume diminishes to between 200 and 500 ml/day. The sodium loss is proportional to the ileostomy volume, so that as the latter falls, so too does the sodium loss which finally reaches between 40 and 60 mmol/day. Any excessive loss is therefore shortlived and relatively easy to manage.

On the other hand, any operation on the gastrointestinal tract involving a breach in the intestine may be followed by a fistula. If a fistula arises from some deep-seated organ, such as the duodenal stump, common bile duct or the tail of the pancreas, it may close providing there is no distal obstruction. However, between the time of establishment of the fistula and its closure, huge quantities of fluid and electrolyte may be lost. A duodenal fistula may discharge all the fluid taken orally together with the swallowed saliva and the gastric, hepatic and pancreatic secretions. Theoretically, even if no oral fluids are given, such as fistula could discharge a volume of fluid in excess of 5 litres/day, which would contain approximately 300 mmol sodium and 90 mmol potassium. However, many surgical fistulae are associated with infection and fever, and this itself will produce a manifold increase in the insensible water loss. A fever of 39°C, with a respiratory rate of 30–40/min may increase the pulmonary water loss from the normal value of 500–750 ml daily up to 2500 ml. In these circumstances, the control of the fluid and electrolyte losses becomes a major feature of postoperative care.

WATER DEPLETION

If the theoretical daily minimum water requirement of 1300 ml is not provided, a pure water depletion occurs. This syndrome is seen most commonly: in the old or extremely ill who are too lethargic to respond to the stimulus of thirst; in patients with lesions of the oesophagus which prevents swallowing; or in patients suffering from a prolonged pyrexia, because sweat is normally hypotonic.

In these circumstances, the urine volume falls rapidly. However, a certain minimum urine volume is required in order to excrete the fixed acids which are formed from protein catabolism. Thus, if the urine volume is insufficient to excrete the solute load, the osmotic pressure of the body fluids increases. In mild cases, the volume deficit falls in both the ECF and the ICF compartments, but as the condition worsens, the secretion of aldosterone produces sodium conservation. This increases the osmolarity of the extracellular fluid and water moves from the intracellular compartment.

Because this syndrome occurs in the apathetic patient, and itself leads to increasing apathy and confusion, there may be delay in recognizing the condition. However, if the patient is secreting negligible quantities of urine, and the plasma sodium concentration is raised above normal (possibly as high as 152 mmol/l), the diagnosis can be assumed. As water depletion becomes worse, the cardiac output begins to fall and respiratory failure may develop.

It is estimated that death due to pure water depletion occurs when about 40% of the initial total body water has been lost. In a 70-kg male, this state could be reached within 13 days.

Treatment

The treatment of water depletion is its replacement, and if this can be achieved by the oral route, so much the better. In the surgical patient who is unconscious, confused or suffering from complete oesophageal obstruction, the fluid must be replaced parenterally. In a conscious patient, the relief of thirst indicates that the condition is improving. In the unconscious patient, improvement is indicated by the increase in urine volume.

WATER INTOXICATION

This is the converse of water depletion. The condition is also known as dilutional hypotonicity or hypotonic overhydration. It arises when more solvent than solute has been administered resulting in the expansion of the fluid compartments which, becoming diluted, also become hypotonic. In the surgical patient, this condition may arise acutely and inadvertently if too great a volume of fluid is administered to a patient unable to excrete it. In the early postoperative period, the intravenous administration of 3–4 litres of 5% glucose in water may be sufficient to induce the symptoms associated with this condition, for during this period abnormal quantities of ADH are suppressing the ability of the kidney to excrete the excess water.

The symptoms of acute water intoxication are normally cerebral: confusion followed by convulsions. Biochemically, the plasma sodium, bicarbonate and chloride concentrations are all depressed. The plasma sodium may reach 105 mmol/l, and an idea of the magnitude of water retention can be gained by realizing that every 3 mmol/l of serum sodium below normal represents, on average, the retention of one litre of water.

Treatment

When the condition has not advanced to the point of convulsions, a patient suffering from water intoxication spontaneously improves if the overloading ceases. The treatment of patients in whom severe neurological symptoms have developed remains a matter for debate. The slow intravenous administration of 5% saline, administering not more than 400 ml in any 24 hours until the acute symptoms have abated was once regarded as the standard treatment, but there are reports especially in the American literature indicating that permanent neurological damage may follow such treatment. Since the majority of cases of water intoxication are iatrogenic, the best treatment is to avoid the condition altogether by restricting the administration of abnormal quantities of fluid during the early postoperative period.

SODIUM DEPLETION

The symptoms and signs of sodium depletion were first described by McCance, in 1936, who found that if sodium was withheld in a test subject the urine became diluted. In this way the body is able to maintain the normal concentration of plasma sodium but at the same time the extracellular fluid volume diminished. He also found that as sodium depletion continued so the plasma sodium level fell, in part due to the movement of this cation into the cells.

The gradual shrinkage of the ECF can be estimated from the haematocrit, since every one-point increase indicates that not only has 100 ml been lost from the plasma but also an additional 400 ml from the interstitial fluid.

Causes of sodium depletion

The surgeon most commonly encounters sodium depletion as a result of intestinal losses. The gastrointestinal fluids are isotonic, except for saliva and the colonic secretions which are hypotonic. Normal saliva and normal stools have an almost identical electrolyte composition with about one-seventh the tonicity of plasma, containing only some 20 mmol/l of anions with a corresponding number of cations as compared to 140 mmol/l in the plasma. However, should an inflammatory or other lesion develop in the colon the fluid secreted becomes more and more like serum moving towards isotonicity.

Symptoms and signs

In any situation, the rate and magnitude of the loss determine the symptomatology.

The loss of large volumes of fluid and salt within a few hours results in clinical shock. Such a situation may be seen in acute gastric dilatation when fluid may be lost at a rate of 1 litre/hour. Because even the grossly dilated stomach can only accommodate 5 litres of fluid, the condition is usually self-limiting unless profuse vomiting occurs; but 5 litres of fluid represents a loss of 30% of the ECF volume, sufficient to produce shock. At the opposite end of the gastrointestinal tract, infection with *Vibrio cholerae* or the development of enterocolitis may lead to the loss of one litre of fluid per hour.

In common surgical conditions such as intestinal obstruction, paralytic ileus and intestinal fistulae it is more common to find that the fluid loss is of the order of 3 l/day. In such states, the peripheral blood pressure may remain normal even when the ECF volume loss is of the order of 30%, but in such patients the CVP may well be zero, in which case the intravascular deficit will be of the order of 700 ml and the interstitial loss 2.8 litres.

In general, a loss of between 300 and 500 mmol of sodium produces clinical evidence of dehydration indicated by the dry mouth, sunken cheeks, furred tongue, loss of skin turgor, thirst and oliguria. Assuming renal function is normal, the scanty output of a highly concentrated urine with an osmolality above 500 mosmols/l and a specific gravity of 1020 or more confirm the diagnosis. The high osmolality of the urine is not due to sodium, because the oliguria is triggered by the volume contraction which in turn leads to excessive secretion of aldosterone. In addition, a pre-renal azotaemia develops, causing a rise in the blood urea nitrogen exceeding the usual 10:1 ratio between blood urea nitrogen and creatinine. Sodium is retained and less than 20 mmol/l will be found in the urine. In this condition, biochemical tests have a limited value since the plasma sodium level does not necessarily indicate the actual sodium loss because of the movement of sodium into the larger intracelluar compartment.

If the condition precipitating the sodium and water loss is allowed to continue, water released by the burning of body fat and the breakdown of protein – 1 g of either releasing 1 ml of water – will be retained, but unfortunately from neither source is salt available. As a result hypotonicity results, but the water needed in the extracellular fluid, because it creates a tonicity gradient between the cellular mass and the extracellular fluid, moves into the cells resulting in cellular swelling. When acute, this causes a host of symptoms due to disturbance of the central nervous system, including disorientation, delirium, convulsions, coma and death.

Treatment

If, when the patient is first seen, there is obvious clinical evidence of dehydration, 4 litres of normal saline each containing 154 mmol of sodium and chloride should be given. Provided the kidneys are normal, the excess chloride can be eliminated. However if the adequacy of renal function is in doubt, a solution containing 154 mmol of sodium should be given with an anion composition of 100 mmol of chloride and 54 mmol of lactate. In this way the possibility of a complicating acidosis is avoided. When the acute crisis is over, the problem of continuing therapy remains. When the volume and electrolyte composition of the fluid loss can be determined, as for example from a pancreatic fistula, the replacement can be 'tailored' to the losses by the addition of solutes to some basic but dilute solution, always remembering that in addition to the losses the normal daily needs of the body should also be met.

The success of any treatment can be judged clinically in many ways: by the improvement in clinical wellbeing, the change to normality of the skin turgor and, especially, by an increasing urine output. The condition can also be monitored in severe cases by measuring the changes taking place in the central venous pressure, the plasma sodium level and the haematocrit.

POTASSIUM

The body contains some 3000–3500 mmol of potassium, 98% of which is within the cells at a concentration of 150 mmol/l. Only 2% of the total body potassium is extracellular, with a concentration between 3.5 and 5.6 mmol/l. Danger lurks at levels below 2.5 and above 7 mmol/l. This potassium gradient is the result of K^+ transport into the cells by NaKATPase and of passive diffusion out of the cells down the K^+ gradient. Both hypo- and hyperkalaemia can produce clinical effects, but normally the loss of total body potassium must exceed 10% of the whole before definite symptoms and signs develop, even though biochemical changes are evident such as a reduced renal excretion. During hypo- or hyperkalaemia, the change in the ECF potassium is proportionally larger than that in the ICF. Both situations lead to alterations in the polarization of the cell membrane, and both tend to produce cardiac arrhythmias.

Potassium depletion

The normal daily intake of potassium is some 100 mmol; this is more than is present in the whole of the extracellular fluid, normally between 40 and 80 mmol. The normal balance of potassium is maintained by the kidneys, but if the body is short of potassium there is no way in which total conservation can be achieved, although its excretion can be decreased by aldosterone antagonists or accelerated by the use of diuretics or aldosterone itself. Thus even in severe depletion states the renal loss continues at some 10 mmol/l of urine passed.

Causes of potassium depletion

The common causes of potassium depletion are losses from the gastrointestinal tract. Interestingly, potassium depletion will not necessarily lead to hypokalaemia, since in the starving patient cellular-destruction with the release of potassium – the catabolic state – feeds the extracellular fluid with potassium. A different set of circumstances exists if the patient is not only deprived of potassium but is also 'stressed', as after major surgery or the complications of surgery. In this situation, hormonal influences lead to greater losses of potassium by the cells. When the loss of potassium is via the gastrointestinal tract, the ultimate biochemical disturbance depends on the site from which this cation is lost. Thus in upper intestinal obstruction, as in pyloric obstruction, the hypokalaemia is associated with alkalosis because of the accompanying chloride loss. In these circumstances, the carbon dioxide concentration rises, and the chloride and potassium concentrations fall. In addition, because the loss of fluid is associated with relatively low concentrations of sodium, a mild degree of sodium depletion also occurs. On the other hand, when the loss of potassium is due to disease of the large bowel, a pure potassium depletion, without an associated alkalosis may develop. The common surgical conditions in which this situation can arise are in ulcerative colitis, by the excessive use of purges and the presence of large villous tumours of the rectum.

As a rule of thumb, a total deficit of 100–200 mmol will lower the serum potassium concentration by about 1 mmol/l. After the initial drop of 1 mmol, higher total losses are required to produce further reduction, about 200–400 mmol for every 1 mmol/l.

Pure potassium depletion may also occur: from renal losses induced by diuretics; by medication with such drugs as carbenoxolone sodium used in the treatment of gastric ulceration; and by the development of aldosterone-secreting tumours of the adrenal cortex, the cause of Conn's syndrome in which the excessive loss of potassium is associated with sodium retention, leading to hypertension.

Symptoms and signs

Severe losses of potassium may be associated with general symptoms such as gradual deterioration of personality, drowsiness and, later, coma. Because hypokalaemia interferes with the normal contractility of smooth, skeletal and cardiac muscle, ileus, generalized weakness and cardiac arrhythmias may occur. Since there is a symbiotic relationship between alkalosis and hypokalaemia, the latter may result in signs of the former causing alkalotic tetany. So far as the heart is concerned, a plethora of abnormalities may appear on the ECG, including ST depression, a prolonged QT interval and inversion of the T wave. If the patient is receiving digitalis, the position is made worse as the effects of potassium depletion summate with the inotropic effects of the former drug, possibly resulting in paroxysmal atrial tachycardia and even partial atrioventricular block.

Chronic hypokalaemia is nephrotoxic, producing vacuolation of the proximal convoluted tubules, hydropic degeneration and diffuse vacuolar degeneration; these changes result in loss of concentrating ability and, in severe prolonged deficiency, interstitial fibrosis and irreversible tubular damage. Thus, in correcting a potassium deficiency, there is a risk that the serum potassium will rise above the toxic level of 7 mmol/l. Therefore the correction of a potassium deficiency should only begin after ensuring that the renal output is adequate, above 20 ml/h. In order to achieve this, a preliminary infusion of 500 ml of 5% glucose solution may be given; as soon as the urine output rises, potassium chloride can be added to the infusion fluid.

Prevention and treatment

To prevent the development of hypokalaemia in the ordinary surgical patient who is receiving intravenous fluids, all that is required is the addition of 40 mmol of KCl to his daily ration. If abnormal losses are occurring these must be added. A patient on nasogastric suction is losing 10–20 mmol of potassium for every litre of fluid aspirated from the stomach.

A patient in whom pure gastric juice is being lost, e.g. the patient suffering from pyloric stenosis, loses not only potassium but also hydrogen ions, and because this causes a disturbance of acid/base balance additional potassium is lost. A patient suffering from a massive villous papilloma of the rectum may lose 200–300 mmol of potassium per litre of the fluid lost.

The treatment of established hypokalaemia is to replace potassium. The safest route of administration is by mouth, giving potassium bicarbonate 1–2 g daily. If this is impossible and the potassium is given intravenously, a large bolus should be avoided since this may cause cardiac problems. Various regimes have been proposed, but the overwhelming consensus is that potassium should not be administered at concentrations above 60 mmol or faster than 60 mmol/h in 5 % glucose, giving a simultaneous injection of 50 units of insulin.

Hyperkalaemia

Whereas the retention of sodium automatically leads to an expansion of the extracellular fluid volume, the retention of potassium is not associated with a similar expansion. The reason there is no corresponding syndrome is due to the high toxicity of potassium. In general, hyperkalaemia is seen by the surgeon only in renal failure, but it is also possible to observe high levels of serum potassium after massive blood transfusions. Although blood has only 3.5 mmol K/litre at the time of collection, this rises to 20–25 mmol/l after two weeks and up to 35 mmol/l by three weeks after collection.

Treatment

As an emergency measure, an almost immediate reduction of a dangerously high potassium level can be achieved by the administration of 250 ml of 25% glucose together with 25 units of insulin given over 4–6 hours, but repetition of such treatment is less successful than its predecessor and after 24 hours there is a danger of hypoglycaemia. Alternatively, ion exchange resins such as polystyrene sulphonate can be given; this insoluble resin exchanges sodium for potassium in the bowel. Every gram of resin exchanges 3 mmol of sodium for potassium. The oral dose is 5–10 g four times daily; the rectal dose, which is more frequently used, is 30 g in 200 ml of a 1% methylcelluose solution every 3–6 hours. These measures are meant to delay the development of toxic symptoms until dialysis can be arranged.

DISTURBANCES OF ACID – BASE BALANCE

Hydrogen ion is produced in great quantities as a byproduct of cellular metabolism. With sugar, insulin and oxygen freely available, sulphuric and phosphoric acid are produced from the breakdown of protein, and lactic, pyruvic and aceto-acetic acid from the incomplete breakdown of sugar and fats. However, only minute concentrations of H^+ ion can be tolerated, the limits compatible with life being between 0.0002 and 0.00012 mmol/l, 20–120 nanomoles per litre, or a pH of between 7.7 and 6.9.

Because the pH values are not linear but a curve – very steep on the side of high H^+ concentrations (smaller pH numbers) and very flat on the side of low pH concentrations (high pH values) – every 0.3 decrease of the pH represents a doubling of the H^+ concentration, whereas every increase of 1 pH unit represents a reduction of the H^+ concentration of one-tenth its former value. Thus, the normal pH of the blood is 7.4; one half the normal concentration, the lowest compatible with life, is represented by a pH of 7.7; and three times the normal, the highest compatible with life, is represented by a pH of 6.9.

Control of acid-base balance

Excluding carbonic acid, 60–100 mmol (60 x 10^6 nmol) of H^+ are produced daily, which is some 100 000 times greater than the total reservoir of H^+ in the extracellular fluid. In order to deal with these vast quantities of H^+ the body uses a series of buffers, the most important of which are bicarbonate and haemoglobin. As the H^+ combines with these materials, so the H^+ concentration in the ECF compartment drops because dissociation takes place only to a limited degree. Blood is a most effective buffer because of its haemoglobin content. If 100 mmol of hydrochloric acid is added to 5 litres of blood, instead of the H^+ concentration rising to the anticipated 20 million nmol (one-half a million times the original value of 40 nmol/l) it will rise to only 80 nmol, double the original. If the intravascular buffers are 'saturated' by an excessive load of H^+, then extracellular and intracellular resources provide additional protection.

As the blood reaches the kidney, hydrogen is extracted from the weak acids and excreted in the urine; the kidney is protected by a further buffering mechanism or by combining the H^+ with ammonia. Thus the kidney is able to excrete all of the 60 million nmol of H^+ produced daily without the urine pH falling below 4.5.

Hydrogen ion is also produced by the dissociation of the weak acid, carbonic acid. Carbon dioxide is a product of cellular metabolism. However, as carbon dioxide is produced, some is immediately combined with water forming carbonic acid while even more is merely dissolved in water. Buffering of the H^+ liberated by carbonic acid is achieved by haemoglobin, and elimination of the dissolved carbon dioxide by the lungs.

Despite use of the terms alkalosis and acidosis to signify changes in the H^+ concentration of the blood, an absolute acidosis, in which the H^+ concentration in the blood exceeds 100 nmol/l, bringing the pH below 7, rarely occurs; whereas alkalosis, in which the concentration of H^+ is depressed below the normal level of around 40 nmol/l with an elevation of the pH above 7.6, is more common.

Causes of acidosis

Acidosis may be produced by:

The excessive production of H^+ ions. This is the cause of acidosis in:

a. Uncontrolled diabetes in which the consumption of fat instead of sugar produces large amounts of fixed acids in the form of ketones.
b. In cellular anoxia following severe shock or in cardiac arrest when, because anaerobic is less effective than aerobic respiration, lactic acid is produced leading to a Type A lactic acidosis.
c. Loss of buffers as in biliary or pancreatic fistulae in which large volumes of alkaline secretions are lost.
d. Failure of pulmonary function, usually seen by the surgeon in patients suffering from severe pulmonary disease in whom respiratory efficiency is still further reduced by an operation, particularly one requiring an incision in the upper abdomen, or by over-sedation because of severe pain.

In all except respiratory failure the condition is classified as 'metabolic acidosis'.

Symptoms and signs

The principle symptoms of severe metabolic acidosis are air hunger together with mental deterioration followed by coma. The severity of the situation can be estimated by measuring the pH, but in order to establish whether the condition is wholly metabolic or in part metabolic and in part respiratory it is also necessary to measure the $P\text{CO}_2$ which is normally 35–45 mmHg (5.4 kPa).

If the pH is 7.1, indicating an increase in H^+ concentration, but the $P\text{CO}_2$ remains within normal limits, this indicates that the increasing number of H^+ ions is not coming from an increase in carbonic acid but must be the result of an increase in unbuffered fixed acids.

Conversely, if the pH is 7.1 but the $P\text{CO}_2$ is 80 mmHg (9.0 kPa) the patient must be suffering from a respiratory acidosis due to inadequate ventilation. The relative contribution of CO_2 and the fixed acids to the overall picture can be calculated from nomograms, which allow one to assess the relative contribution of carbonic and fixed acids and also indicate what part the lung is playing in an attempt to ameliorate the acidotic state.

Treatment of acidosis

The majority of patients suffering from chronic renal or pulmonary disease live with a mild but steady-state degree of imbalance; for them no treatment is required and, indeed, may be valueless. Since acute disturbances of the acid – base balance are always secondary to some underlying cause, no long-term cure can result from the treatment of the imbalance itself; the underlying cause must, if possible, be brought under control.

Respiratory acidosis

Respiratory acidosis is most commonly seen by the surgeon in individuals suffering from poor pulmonary function in whom an upper abdominal incision is required, in patients suffering from a chest injury or following over-sedation. In these circumstances some form of mechanical ventilation may be required. The kidney attempts to correct the acidotic state by increasing the tubular reabsorption of sodium and bicarbonate, and increasing the excretion of hydrogen and ammonium ions. Another important aspect of respiratory acidosis is the potential for dangerous levels of hyperkalaemia to develop. This is produced by the rise in H^+ ion concentration in the plasma causing a movement of this ion into the cells in exchange for potassium, producing a potential hyperkalaemia which is reversed as the acidosis is corrected. However, if the acidotic state persists for some time, the excess K^+ ions are excreted by the kidney so that, if the acidosis is rapidly corrected, as the H^+ ion leaves the cell to be replaced by K^+ ion a sudden fall in the serum potassium occurs. Changes in the potassium level should therefore be carefully monitored, and potassium administered if dangerous levels of hypokalaemia develop.

Metabolic acidosis

In metabolic acidosis the underlying disorder must be corrected if this is possible, and the H^+ ion concentration must be reduced. The lungs play their part because the increase in the rate and depth of respiration leads to a reduction in carbonic acid. However, beyond a base deficit of 6 mmol/l (equivalent to a bicarbonate value of 22 mmol/l), complete respiratory compensation is impossible. Theoretically, H^+ ion could be removed by continuous gastric suction, a nasogastric tube being positioned in the stomach, gastric secretion stimulated by the administration of pentagastrin and the highly acid gastric juice aspirated. However, the chief tool used in the correction of a metabolic acidosis is the administration of bicarbonate. The theoretical amount required in a given situation can be calculated by measuring the bicarbonate content of the blood, and by multiplying the defect by the volume of extracellular fluid to arrive at the number of mmol of bicarbonate required. Thus, considering the normal bicarbonate to be 24 mmol/l and the normal extracellular fluid volume to be 14 litres, if the reported bicarbonate level is 14 mmol/l the approximate extracellular defect of bicarbonate is 140 mmol. Theoretically there should be added to this figure the deficit of other extracellular buffers and the intracellular buffers which are regenerated at the expense of the administered bicarbonate. However, assuming adequate rehydration and the control of the underlying condition, the safest way to administer bicarbonate is by considering only the extracellular defect.

In an emergency, an infusion of 8.4% sodium bicarbonate can be administered intravenously at a rate of 0.1 mmol/kg per minute, not more than 50 ml being given before re-estimating the $Pa\text{CO}_2$ and the pH. In the surgical patient, a 'mixed' acidosis is nearly always associated with a marked reduction in the ECF as a result of intestinal losses. In such patients, an infusion of normal or half-normal saline should either precede or immediately follow the administration of bicarbonate. Clinically, the relief of metabolic acidosis can be judged by the decrease in 'air hunger'.

Alkalosis

Metabolic alkalosis

The commonest cause of a metabolic alkalosis is the uninhibited vomiting of patients suffering from pyloric stenosis. However, if this condition remains untreated by surgery it becomes complicated by the additional loss of both sodium and potassium, with the result that the simple administration of ammonium chloride is inadequate to correct the metabolic defect. A further difficulty is that of measuring the magnitude of the total body deficit of potassium, which may be considerable if the patient has been vomiting for a prolonged period. Clinically, severe alkalosis is associated with phasic respiration and tetany, because as the pH rises so too does the plasma bicarbonate level. The pH of the urine is also high and the urine urea may be low despite a high blood urea.

To correct the condition, the potassium depletion is first repaired before the administration of sodium or ammonium chloride. This is achieved by intravenous potassium chloride, giving not more than 10 mmol/h in a severe alkalotic state. Since the potassium deficiency may be equal to one-third the total body potassium, there is little need to fear the cardiac effects of potassium toxicity so long as renal function is normal or is expected to be normal when the extracellular fluid volume has been replaced with normal saline.

Respiratory alkalosis

Normally a product of overbreathing, this condition is usually treated by sedation.

11 Diabetes and the surgeon

Diabetes affects approximately 10 per 1000 of the population. It is a metabolic disorder of importance to the surgeon in a number of respects.

1. The disease impairs some of the mechanisms which would normally act to preserve homeostasis during and after operative stress. As a result the patient is more sensitive to protein depletion, depletion or excess of sugar and disturbances of salt and water metabolism. The chief metabolic danger of unrecognized diabetes, however, is the possibility of severe unrecognized hypoglycaemia or, alternatively, severe ketoacidosis following surgery.
2. If diabetes is uncontrolled, there is a greater tendency to infection. Although a normal polymorphonuclear leucocytosis occurs, the phagocytic activity of the leucocytes, falls possibly due to the osmotic pressure of the exudate. Furthermore, when diabetes is uncontrolled there is a tendency for an overgrowth of microorganisms. For example, in the female, mucocutaneous candidiasis of the vulva occurs more commonly than in the normal woman. In either sex there is an increased incidence of non-clostridial gas-forming infections in surgical wounds. In ketoacidosis, granulocyte mobilization is impaired both systematically and locally around an infected area, accompanied by a decreased phagocytic function. However, the well-controlled diabetic is no more susceptible to infection than a normal individual.
3. However well-controlled, diabetes is associated with small vessel disease which leads to decreased peripheral perfusion and a tendency to develop infections with microaerophilic or anaerobic organisms.
4. Neuropathy leads to trophic ulceration of the feet which may

precipitate gangrene or, affecting the bladder, lead to the retention of urine.

So far as the surgeon is concerned, the patient may be admitted to his care as a known diabetic. Under these circumstances, the severity of the metabolic derangement can be assessed from the following facts.

1. The age of onset of the disease. The young diabetic is almost always insulin-dependent and may be 'fragile', i.e. psychologically incapable of controlling his own disease, or 'brittle', i.e. he or she may have frequent attacks of ketoacidosis.
2. The therapeutic requirements of the patient. If the dose of insulin required to control the disease exceeds 40 units, the disease is of moderate severity and potentially such a patient may develop a severe postoperative imbalance.

MANAGEMENT OF THE DIABETIC PATIENT: GENERAL PRINCIPLES

The state of the diabetic condition should be established on admission. This can easily be achieved in 24 hours, and if the operation is 'elective' and repeated blood sugars show that the disease is poorly controlled, the operation should be postponed. If on the other hand it is shown to be well-controlled, the operation can proceed, preferably placing the patient first on the list in the morning.

If the patient is admitted as a surgical emergency and not in a state of ketoacidosis, no time should be lost in establishing the degree of stability and the operation should be performed. However if the patient is admitted in a state of ketoacidosis, this should be controlled, especially as it itself might be the cause of the 'acute abdomen'. The agents now used for the control of diabetes are as follows:

1. Diet

It is now customary to use a carbohydrate-restricted diet and, in the absence of obesity, a carbohydrate intake of between 100 and 250 g is usually allowed, much depending on the patient's work. The overall amount of fat and protein allowed is dependent only on the presence or absence of obesity.

2. Oral hypoglycaemic agents

These are divisible into two groups: the sulphonylurea compounds and the biguanides. The first group includes the drugs chlorpropamide, with a daily dose of 0.1–0.5 g, and tolbutamide, daily dose 1–6 g daily. These compounds act by stimulating the release of insulin from the pancreas; in addition they have some action on the liver, inhibiting glucose output and increasing the deposition of glycogen. Chlorpropamide is unique in that it has a long half-life and is excreted extremely slowly, factors which allow it to be used in a single daily dose. These agents are ineffective in insulin-dependent juvenile diabetics and usually give the best results in non-ketotic asymptomatic diabetics over 40 years of age whose insulin requirements are less than 40 units. The most commonly used biguanide is phenformin which is best used in patients with a high insulin requirement. Biguanides do not stimulate the release of insulin from the islet cells but supplement the effects of insulin on the peripheral utilization of glucose. The duration of action of phenformin is 6–8 hours but, using a time-delayed capsule, as little as 50 mg twice daily may suffice. Both groups of drugs may cause gastrointestinal upset. By the skilful use of diet, 50% of diabetics can now be controlled by oral hypoglycaemic agents alone.

3. Naturally-occurring insulin

The active principle controlling diabetes was first isolated by Banting and Best in 1922. Insulin is a polypeptide which is normally liberated from the islet cells in response to glucose and the insulin level in the blood. Soluble unmodified insulin has a 'start' time of one hour, a maximal effect of 2–3 hours and a lasting effect of 8 hours. For this reason, various combinations have been produced, mainly combining insulin with protamine and zinc, in order to prolong the time of action. One combination in common use is Isophane Insulin Injection B.P. which contains a zinc insulin modified by protamine. It may contain 40 or 80 units of insulin per millilitre. Its blood sugar lowering action is intermediate between that of Protamine Zinc Insulin and Globin Zinc Insulin. The onset of its action is 1–2 hours and peak activity is reached 10–20 hours later. An average diabetic may well be sustained on 20 units of soluble insulin and 30 units of isophane, both injections being given in the morning.

Conventional insulin may be separated into: component a,

a material of high molecular weight; component b, comprising pro-insulin, intermediates and a dimer; and component c, comprising insulin, arginine insulin, the ethylester of insulin and deamidoinsulin. The development of antibodies and fat dystrophy are believed to be associated with contaminant materials, but it is also agreed that component a is antigenic as also are components b and c. This has led to the development of insulin structurally identical to human insulin produced either by the chemical manipulation of insulin from animal sources or by the use of recombinant DNA technology; such insulins are known as 'human insulins'. These types of insulin are indicated in patients who develop fat dystrophy or become insulin-resistant, but there is little indication for their use when a patient is stable and well-controlled or ordinary insulin.

MANAGEMENT OF THE DIABETIC THROUGHOUT AN OPERATION OF MODERATE SEVERITY

The following assumptions are made:

1. The operation is elective and the patient is a moderately severe diabetic requiring 40 units of insulin per day.
2. Blood sugar and urine estimations over a 24-hour period preoperatively have shown that he is well balanced.

Treatment

One-half of the patient's daily insulin requirement is given on the morning of the operation and an intravenous drip of 10% glucose in water is commenced. Assuming that the operation lasts for one hour, the patient is controlled during the remainder of the day by blood sugar estimations performed at 2-hourly intervals. Throughout the day, some 200–400 g of glucose should be given in 2–3000 ml of fluid. If the blood sugar is less than 5.5 mmol/l, no soluble insulin is administered; if it is 8.25 mmol/l, 8 units are administered; if 8.25–11.0 mol/l, 12 units; and 11–16 mmol/l, 16 units. If, however, the blood sugar has risen to 16 mmol/l or more, there is urgent need for an estimation of the electrolytes, including pH and CO_2-combining power, since the patient is probably approaching ketosis.

On the day following the operation, administration of soluble insulin should be continued. Assuming that the patient is able to take fluids by mouth and an intravenous drip of 5% glucose is in situ, urine testing with a Clinitest tablet, rather than blood levels, should be used for estimating the requirements of soluble insulin. The method is as follows. If the tablet placed in 5 drops of urine and 10 drops of water changes to blue, no insulin is required. A change to green indicates 0.5% sugar in which case 8 units of insulin are required; and a change to brown, indicating 1% sugar, requires 12 units. Finally, an orange discolouration indicates 2% sugar and a need for 16 units of soluble insulin together with investigation to exclude developing ketosis. If no problems arise and the patient is having no gastrointestinal difficulties, he may return to his regular schedule on the second postoperative day.

If the patient is controlled by diet and an oral hypoglycaemic agent alone, the dose of the oral agent should be converted into its insulin equivalent. Thus, 250 mg of chlorpropamide are equivalent to 25 units of soluble insulin, 75–100 mg phenformin to 15 units of insulin, and 1500 mg of tolbutamide, 15 units. The conversion is performed and, as above, one-half of the daily requirement in the form of soluble insulin is given on the morning of the operation.

MANAGEMENT OF THE DIABETIC ADMITTED IN KETOACIDOSIS

If the patient is admitted as an acute surgical emergency suffering from diabetic ketoacidosis, even if the primary cause of the emergency appears to be general peritonitis, the treatment of the metabolic imbalance takes priority in order of treatment. A diabetic coma may develop with dramatic suddeness when the imbalance is caused by infection. The patient appears dehydrated, the breath smells of acetone and respiration is laboured. The urine usually contains large amounts of sugar and acetoacetic acid, the blood pressure falls and there is a weak, rapid pulse. Finally, coma develops, although the depth of coma bears no relationship to the changes in the extracellular fluid.

Ketones in the urine are detected by the use of a Labstix, the shade of lavender or purple at 15 seconds indicating the concentration. Once the condition begins, it is 'fed' by the breakdown of tissue protein which results in the liberation of ketogenic amino acids, such as leucine, phenylalanine and tyrosine. In severe cases, 20% of the body water may be lost, due in part to the precipitating cause and in part to the ketogenic state itself. Sodium loss of the order of 500 mmol may occur due to its excretion in the urine with acetoacetic acid. Vomiting accelerates the dehydration.

Although on the initial investigation of the electrolyte concentrations the plasma potassium may be elevated, there is a severe potassium deficit, due in part to vomiting and in part to renal excretion. As the patient becomes more acidotic, an increasing amount of sodium is taken up by the acetoacetic acid leaving the bicarbonate ion in isolation; the deep sighing respiration known as Kussmaul's breathing represents an attempt to get rid of the excess carbon dioxide and restore the normal plasma ration of bicarbonate to carbon dioxide of 20:1. The CO_2-combining power therefore falls below the normal level of 22–26 mmol/l, and the pH falls below the normal value of 7.4.

The immediate investigations required in these circumstances are an estimation of the blood sugar, serum sodium, potassium, chloride, pH and P_{CO_2} and, if possible, a measurement of the serum lactic acid.

Treatment

An immediate intravenous infusion of normal saline is commenced, with the object of giving the first litre in one hour. In addition, 40 units of soluble insulin are given. As a rule of thumb, 10 units of insulin should decrease the blood sugar by 5.5 mmol/l, unless the patient is insulin-resistant. At the end of the first hour, the infusion of a further litre of normal saline in 5% glucose is commenced and the estimations are repeated. If the blood sugar remains unaltered, a further 80 units of soluble insulin are given. If the blood sugar has fallen by less than half, a further 40 units are administered; if by more than half, 20 units. If, on the second estimation, the serum potassium has fallen to apparently normal levels, between 40 and 80 mmol should be added to the infusion fluid. This must not, however, be given if the patient is azotaemic, oliguric or anuric. If the pH is grossly disturbed, say below 7.1, 100 mmol of sodium bicarbonate should be added to the transfusion. Below 6.9, 200 mmol may be necessary.

Correction or near correction may be achieved within three hours. If the cause of the abdominal pain was the ketoacidosis itself, it will have improved within this period making operation unwarranted.

Prior to the induction of anaesthesia, 20 g of glucose together with 20 units of soluble insulin should be given. Throughout anaesthesia, the serum glucose and pH, together with the $P\text{CO}_2$, should be monitored at frequent intervals.

Another form of coma which may occur is known as hyperos-molar non-ketoacidosis. This is occasionally seen in diabetics whose disease begins in middle-age. An infection may precipitate the condition, but the symptoms are usually of gradual onset and are associated with extremely high blood glucose concentrations. There is no marked acidosis and the condition is treated by the administration of large amounts of water, insulin and potassium; the latter is especially important since death may occur from hypokalaemia.

The author recognizes that many other regimes have been described for the treatment of diabetes and of its major complication of ketosis. All that has been attempted here is to lay down principles which, if followed, will be of benefit and will allow one time to consult one's medical colleagues.

12 Assessment of cardiopulmonary function in the pre- and postoperative patient

HISTORY

The first step in the assessment of cardiopulmonary function in the preoperative patient is to obtain a clear and adequate history of past medical complaints and social habits.

Among the most significant social habits about which information is required is the patient's attitude to smoking. This is one of the three identifiable aetiological factors related to the development of chronic bronchitis and emphysema, the other two being atmospheric pollution and infection.

Smoking. The incidence of chronic bronchitis – defined as a condition in which sputum is coughed up on most days for at least three consecutive months in two successive years – is some four times greater in heavy smokers as compared to non-smokers, being of the order of 20% in the former as compared to 5% in the latter. In keeping with this finding, simple tests of respiratory function show that smokers have a reduced FEV_1 and diffusing capacity as compared to non-smokers.

These changes are the result of the numerous pathological changes induced by smoking, which include:

1. Mucosal gland hypertrophy which causes an increase in secretion.
2. Inhibition of the bronchial ciliary blanket.

These two factors acting together predispose to the accumulation of mucus in the bronchial tree as a result of which an increased liability to infection follows. In addition, both macrophages and neutrophil leucocytes accumulate, the latter releasing elastase and both together causing the local inactivation of alpha-antitrypsin-releasing oxidants.

The protease and anti-protease imbalance resulting from these changes is thought to be the cause of the emphysema so frequently found in association with chronic bronchitis; this emphysema with its associated loss of lung supporting substance makes a major contribution to airway obstruction.

Atmospheric pollution is also of great importance. Indeed, it is considered that the Clean Air Acts of recent years have had a considerable influence not only in reducing the incidence of chronic pulmonary disease but also in reducing the volume of sputum associated with the disease when it occurs.

Infection. The role of childhood infection has also been recognized as a possible cause of chronic pulmonary disease in later life, although it is admitted that the cause may not be the infection as such but, rather, the poor social conditions in which such infants live.

The ultimate functional result of these changes is airway obstruction brought about by a variable combination of: excessive mucus in the lumen of the airways; thickening of the bronchial mucus membranes; increased bronchial muscle tone; increased collapsibility of the peripheral airways due to loss of cartilage and loss of lung retractive forces due to emphysema; and invagination of the soft posterior wall of the larger bronchi and trachea on expiration caused by the steep gradient between the extrabronchial and intraluminal pressures.

PHYSICAL TYPES

In the 'full blown' clinical picture, two types of patient have been described:

1. The 'blue bloater' who is suffering from chronic bronchitis is often short, stocky and commonly cyanosed.
2. The 'pink puffer' who is purely emphysematous and is often asthenic.

In the typical chronic bronchitic, the characteristic symptoms are a wheeze, productive cough and breathlessness. As the condition progresses, so the cough persists for longer periods and becomes progressively more productive, occurring not only in the morning but throughout the day and even keeping the affected individual awake at night, particularly as a coughing attack will frequently follow a change in position. Patients suffering from chronic bronchitis find that mild upper respiratory infections of little significance in the normal individual rapidly affect the chest, causing increasing volumes of sputum which will alter in colour as infection is established.

At the other end of the spectrum, in the purely emphysematous patient, the cough, sputum and wheeze appear relatively unimportant. The principle disabling feature is breathlessness and often a progressive dyspnoea which frequently begins after an apparently mild chest infection. This latter type of patient sits expiring slowly with the lips pursed in order to raise the intrapulmonary pressure and so prevent the collapse of his thin-walled bronchioles.

In the majority of patients, the condition is a mixture of the two and in the end stage, right-sided heart failure occurs secondary to pulmonary hypertension brought about by an acute respiratory infection.

PHYSICAL EXAMINATION

This may reveal cynasis, but the most common physical sign on inspection is the use made by the patient of the accessory muscles of respiration, with possible indrawing of the suprasternal, supraclavicular fossae and the intercostal muscles. In addition, the jugular veins may be congested. In severe airway obstruction, the patient may have to raise the intrathoracic pressure above the atmospheric pressure in order to expire. This causes the jugular pressure to rise on expiration, falling back on inspiration, but if the latter does not occur the patient is suffering from cardiac failure.

Percussion may reveal a decrease in the area of cardiac and hepatic dullness, indicating the degree to which the lungs are hyperinflated or emphysematous.

On auscultation, the most common finding is generalized wheezing across the whole chest, most often expiratory but frequently inspiratory. In addition, the breath sounds may have a prolonged expiratory phase or be uniformly diminished; the decrease, if present, correlates well with the degree of airway obstruction.

CLINICAL CONSEQUENCES OF CHRONIC CHEST DISEASE IN THE SURGICAL PATIENT

In general terms, mild degrees of chronic bronchitis and emphysema are relatively unimportant in the young patient as regards mortality but may contribute to an increase in post-surgical morbidity by increasing the incidence of wound haematomata and wound dehiscence. In older patients, however, the postoperative reduction of pulmonary function which occurs especially following upper abdominal incisions – when the total lung capacity has been shown to be reduced by as much as 2.4 litres and the peak respiratory flow (PRF) by as much as 50% – may be sufficient to precipitate death from respiratory failure.

PREOPERATIVE ASSESSMENT OF A PATIENT COMPLAINING OF A CHRONIC COUGH

Unless a patient is complaining of pulmonary disease, routine chest X-rays are of little use; indeed, the Royal College of Radiologists in 1979 regarded routine chest X-rays as of no value since they had no influence on operative morbidity, a minimal yield of unsuspected clinical abnormalities and a negligible effect on patient management. Even in patients with an appreciable disability from chronic bronchitis and emphysema, little may be seen on a plain postero-anterior chest radiograph.

In severe disease the peripheral vascular shadows may be thinned, straightened or lost as the vessels are deranged by advancing disease, the diaphragm appears flattened and the posterior ends of the 11th and 12th ribs may be visible. On a lateral projection, overdistension of the lungs may be indicated by the large retrosternal airspace; 3 cm below the manubrium the horizontal distance from the posterior surface of the aorta to the sternum may exceed 4.5 cm.

Functional tests

The functional tests of greatest value in assessing pulmonary function in the preoperative patient need to be simple and easy to execute. A test commonly used is the forced expiratory volume in one second FEV_1. The peak flow is simply measured using a Wright's peak flow meter. The blood gases, are only necessary if the FEV_1 is less than 50% of the predicted value, as obtained from nomograms which relate these values to age, sex and height. In considering peak flow rates, values up to 100 l/min less than the predicted are regarded as normal in men, and in women values less than 85 l/min. All tests of respiratory function except blood gas analyses require the cooperation of the patient, and the definitive measurement is usually made after one or two practice attempts.

Another common routine test is a measurement of the forced vital capacity (FVC) with the result expressed as the FEV_1 and also as a percentage of the vital capacity. If the FEV_1/FVC ratio is 80% or better it is considered normal, but if the ratio is below 60% every effort should be made to obtain some improvement before surgery.

Nunn and his coworkers examined the postoperative course of a group of patients suffering from severe chronic obstructive pulmonary disease, who were all dyspnoeic on exertion and in whom the majority suffered from a chronic productive cough, and the minority, unrelenting dyspnoea. They found that the FEV_1 was a good preoperative screening test supplemented by arterial blood gases when the FEV_1 had fallen to less than 1 litre. The commonest routine test was a measurement of the forced vital capacity with the result expressed as the FEV_1 and also as a percentage of the slow vital capacity.

As a result of his investigations, Nunn was able to divide the patients into three groups.

Group I. Those patients with a low FEV_1 but with a normal $Pa\text{CO}_2$ without overt hypoxaemia, $Pa\text{O}_2$ greater than 7.3 kPa (55 mmHg).
Group II. Those patients with a low FEV_1 and a low $Pa\text{O}_2$ of less than 7.3 kPa but a normal $Pa\text{CO}_2$.
Group III. Those patients with a greatly reduced FEV_1 and a $Pa\text{CO}_2$ greater than 5.9 kPa (44 mmHg) in whom there was also overt hypoxaemia with the $Pa\text{O}_2$ of less than 7.3 kPa.

In the first group, little was required in the way of respiratory support following operation; however Group II patients all required prolonged O_2 administration in the postoperative period, and in Group III full ventilatory support was required.

Nunn therefore concluded that a reduced FEV_1 without hyercapnia or hypoxia was no barrier to routine surgery, but that values below 1 litre or a reduction of 50% required careful monitoring following operation. He concluded that the most important laboratory measurement in preoperative assessment was a raised $Pa\text{CO}_2$, an increase above 6.7 kPa (50 mmHg) indicating the need for postoperative artificial ventilation and possibly prolonged endotracheal intubation. Nevertheless, the finding of abnormal respiratory function, especially when associated with sputum production, is an indication to pursue a course of preoperative physiotherapy combined with postural drainage, antibiotics if the sputum is infected and a test of bronchodilator drugs.

RESPIRATORY FAILURE

Respiratory failure is a condition in which the lungs fail to oxygenate adequately the arterial blood and/or fail to prevent CO_2 retention. There is no absolute definition of the levels of PaO_2 and $PaCO_2$ which indicate respiratory failure. As a general guide, a PaO_2 of less than 60 mmHg (7.09 kPa) or a $PaCO_2$ of more than 50 mmHg (6.74 kPa) are figures accepted by most surgeons but, in practice, the significance of such values depends considerably on the past history of the patient.

The hypoxaemia of respiratory failure after surgery is usually caused by a combination of the following four mechanisms: hypoventilation, diffusion impairment, and shunt and ventilation/perfusion inequality. Ventilation/perfusion inequality is by far the most important, and is largely responsible for the low PO_2 complicating obstructive airway disease, in which, postoperatively, the added feature of hypoventilation occurs due to pain and sedation, especially after upper abdominal incisions.

The signs of hypoxaemia when the arterial PO_2 rapidly drops to levels between 40 and 50 mmHg are cyanosis, tachycardia, mental clouding and, if there is associated coronary artery disease, heart failure, But in nearly all surgical patients, the condition and its severity are determined by serial PaO_2 measurements following surgery, rather than by the recognition of the above symptoms.

The significance of hypoxaemia rests on the fact that it results in immediate tissue anoxia, although the various tissues of the body vary considerably in their vulnerability. Thus, at greatest risk is the central nervous system, in which a complete cessation of blood leads to a loss of consciousness within 10–20 secs, and complete irreversible changes occur within 3–5 minutes.

If the PO_2 falls below a critical level in the tissues, aerobic is replaced by anaerobic glycolysis, with the formation of increasing levels of lactic acid. Anaerobic glycolysis is a relatively inefficient method of obtaining energy from glucose, but nevertheless plays a critical role in maintaining tissue viability in respiratory failure. The large amounts of lactic acid released into the blood cause a metabolic acidosis but, when tissue oxygenation is improved, the lactic acid can be reconverted to glucose and used directly for energy; the greater part of this conversion taking place in the liver.

Carbon dioxide retention resulting in hypercapnia occurs as a result of a combination of hypoventilation and ventilation/perfusion inequality, the latter being the important factor in patients suffering from chronic obstructive airway disease. It can also be caused by the injudicious use of oxygen therapy, since – like patients suffering from chronic uraemia who can live comfortably on a relatively low haemoglobin and high creatinine level – the patient suffering from chronic pulmonary disease can live with severe hypoxaemia and a degree of hypercapnia which would be unsustainable when occurring acutely. In such patients, the ventilatory drive, which requires a high workload of breathing, comes from the hypoxic stimulation of the peripheral chemoreceptors. If a mild upper respiratory tract infection should then occur and be treated with a high inspired oxygen concentration, the hypoxic ventilatory drive is abolished whilst the work of breathing is increased due to the retention of secretions with the possible overlay of bronchospasm. As a result, ventilation is depressed and very high levels of arterial $PaCO_2$ may develop followed by the rapid onset of profound hypoxaemia if the oxygen is discontinued.

Respiratory failure is divided into types I and II. In type I, hypoxia without hypercapnia occurs due to ventilation/perfusion imbalance, venous admixture and alveolar capillary block, the first of these factors being the most important in the respiratory failure seen in the surgical patient. The treatment of such a patient is by administration of high concentrations of oxygen together with treatment of the underlying disease.

In type II respiratory failure, both hypoxaemia and hypercapnia occur. In the surgical patient, this type of acute respiratory failure may follow acute receptor failure when a chronic bronchitic is subjected to abdominal surgery or suffers a chest injury. In this type of patient, the oxygen therapy should be so controlled that the hypoxia is relieved without allowing increasing hypercapnia and acidosis to develop. Regular checks of the blood gases and the pH are required for such control, measuring in particular the $PaCO_2$, which should be maintained above 6.6 kPa (50 mmHg); the pH should be above 7.25. If these levels cannot be achieved by using nasal cannulae or masks with the administration of respiratory stimulants such as doxopram 15 mg/min by continous intravenous transfusion, artificial ventilation must be considered.

Artificial ventilation

When artificial ventilation is used, the complete control of the inspired gases is automatically achieved. At present, tracheostomy is avoided and endotracheal intubation using a nasotracheal tube is the preferred method. The cuff should be inflated to the lowest acceptable pressure and it should be periodically deflated and changed every three days. Several types of assisted ventilation are available depending to some extent on the individual physician's choice.

In general terms, a chronic bronchitic passing into acute respiratory failure following surgery will be placed on continous mandatory ventilation (CMV). This will be continued for 24–48 hours and then replaced by synchronous intermittent mandatory ventilation (SIMV), in which the patient initiates the inspiratory effort, but if this does not provide sufficient ventilation to overcome the anoxia, the ventilator itself can be set to provide an adequate minute volume.

If collapse of distal segments of the respiratory tree are present, e.g. in collapse following surgery, either continuous positive airway pressure (CPAP) or positive end expiratory pressure (PEEP) can be used although using the latter the patient must be sedated and paralysed.

Weaning

The criteria needed for weaning are similar to those used for ventilatory support. The chief factors concerned are whether:

a. The patient can breath spontaneously.
b. gas exchange is adequate.
c. the patient can cough, and so clear the bronchial tree.
d. the tidal volume is adequate.
e. a normal $Pa\text{CO}_2$ can be preserved.

In some patients – particularly those in whom severe chronic pulmonary disease is already present prior to the precipitating factor causing pulmonary failure – slow, careful weaning from the ventilator may be necessary, weaning for an interval and then reverting to it for another period. This process may require some days. In patients with no previous history of chronic pulmonary disease such measures may be unnecessary.

CARDIAC DISEASE AND HYPERTENSION

There can be little doubt that a diseased heart is more vulnerable to the strains of major surgery than one which is completely healthy, but the published data make a precise assessment of the increased risk difficult to evaluate because of the wide differences of opinion expressed. However, a patient in whom the myocardium is diseased but functional compensation is complete is at minimal risk, even after major surgery. The risk is also minimal in the patient suffering from moderate hypertension, although such patients are subject to marked haemodynamic responses to both anaesthesia and surgery.

A severe uncontrolled rise in the blood pressure in a hypertensive, atherosclerotic individual may lead to a cerebrovascular accident or, by increasing the workload of the heart, left ventricular failure, a rise in the left ventricular end diastolic pressure and, possibly pulmonary oedema. If the intramural coronary arteries have been affected with atheroma, a raised diastolic blood pressure may jeopardize myocardial bloodflow, producing changes in the ECG. As might be expected, 'malignant' hypertension – the term being applied to patients with a diastolic blood pressure of 120 mmHg (16.3 kPa) or more, together with papilloedema and lesions of the arterioles, in whom a known aetiological factor can be identified – is associated with a much higher mortality following surgery than is the more common 'essential' hypertension. Thus, if a patient is admitted and found to be hypertensive, surgery should be delayed until the hypertension is brought under control by diuretics and/or β-blockers. If emergency surgery is required in an untreated hypertensive patient, some protection can be afforded by the intravenous administration of 0.025–0.1 mg/kg of the β-blocker, propranolol.

If a patient has suffered a myocardial infarction less than three months prior to operation, a relatively high mortality can be expected. The site of the infarct is of some importance, subendocardial lesions being associated with a lesser mortality than those which are transmural. After three months, although the mortality may be slightly higher than in a normal healthy person, the infarct will have healed and there is little point in delaying operation. However, it is recommended that patients who have suffered a major infarct should be given tranquillizing drugs prior to surgery in order to allay the natural anxiety normally felt preoperatively, and that during operation especial care should be taken to avoid hypoxia and excessive changes in the blood pressure.

If a patient has a history of rheumatic endocarditis, is a victim of congenital cardiac abnormalities or has been the recipient of artificial heart valves, the administration of antibiotics preoperatively and during the course of the postoperative period is essential to avoid the dangers associated with subacute bacterial endocarditis or infection of the valves.

In general, therefore, the surgical indications for a particular operation take precedence over the cardiac condition. If the heart is decompensating or decompensated, time should be taken to treat the patient until maximal improvement of the cardiorespiratory system has been achieved, if the operation is not urgent. If the heart is decompensating, the symptoms are fatigue and dyspnoea on exertion. Nocturnal dyspnoea – cardiac asthma – develops somewhat later and is due to pulmonary congestion followed by oedema, and death may occur with great rapidity. In the majority of patients, however, both sides of the heart fail, with the production of congestive heart failure. All the symptoms described may be present, and examination may reveal an increase in the size of the heart. Size is, however, dependent on the ability of the myocardium to hypertrophy and dilate. In the elderly, the ischaemic myocardium may be so fibrotic that it cannot hypertrophy. Disturbances of rhythm, engorgement of the neck veins, crepitations at the lung bases, enlargement of the liver, ascites and dependent oedema may all be evident. In this condition, the patient is clearly unfit for surgery, but some improvement can be achieved even in a few hours, because the drugs used to aid a failing heart take only a short time to exert their effect.

The commonest medicinal preparation used in the treatment of cardiac failure is digitalis or one of its many derivatives. These have three fundamental actions on the heart: they increase the contractile force, and alter myocardial excitability and conductivity, thereby affecting cardiac rhythm. The administration of digitalis is indicated when damage to the myocardium has led to decompensation but these drugs are also administered in auricular fibrillation when the ventricular rate may be slowed from 130–150 b.p.m. down to 50–60 b.p.m. in the course of a few hours. In approximately one-half of patients suffering from atrial flutter, normal sinus rhythm can be achieved without the use of other drugs. The use of digitalis in paroxysmal atrial tachycardia is only indicated if the condition does not respond to simple vagal stimulation produced by pressure on the carotid sinus or, alternatively, to neostigmine 0.5 mg subcutaneously.

Rarely, death can occur from digitalis overdosage. Usually, a warning in the form of vomiting occurs as a result of overdosage, but severe cerebral effects may also occur as can almost any kind of cardiac arrhythmia due to derangements of the conducting system.

If rapid digitalization is required, the most commonly used preparation is digoxin, 0.5–1.0 mg being given slowly intravenously. The action of digoxin begins within a few minutes and reaches its maximal effect within five hours. The normal duration of action is 4–7 days. The usual maintenance dose of digoxin is 0.25–0.75 mg daily. The only absolute contraindication to the use of digitalis is the presence of ventricular ectopic rhythms; relative contraindications include hypokalaemia and partial atrioventricular block.

Congestive heart failure is associated with retention of sodium and water, and diuretics are required to remove this overload. A drug such as chlorothiazide, 0.5–2.0 mg daily by mouth, may be given, noting that this will not only rid the body of excess water but also promote the concomitant loss of potassium which must be replaced by giving potassium chloride or bicarbonate.

If the patient has been digitalized, and is taking diuretics at the time of admission to hospital for emergency or elective surgery, the drugs will need to be continued after operation by oral or parenteral administration, whichever is more appropriate. When the operation is elective, a few days in hospital, giving time for assessment of the cardiopulmonary system, may be of great benefit to a patient in the postoperative period.

Occasionally, a patient suffering from compensated heart disease suddenly develops a paroxysm of left-sided failure. Pulmonary congestion develops followed by oedema and crepitations at both bases and the patient becomes critically ill. The 'first aid' treatment of this condition is to prop the patient up immediately so as to lower the central venous pressure. Morphine sulphate 5–10 mg intravenously depresses purposeless stimulation of the respiratory centre, and aminophylline 0.5 g by slow intravenous injection relieves the associated bronchospasm, diminishes the venous pressure and increases cardiac rate. In addition, the rapidly acting diuretic, frusemide, 40 mg intravenously, should be administered and the patient should be given oxygen.

In the postoperative period, the surgeon should always remember than when a previously asymptomatic patient develops sudden chest pain of anginal type, it may indicate occult haemorrhage which has so increased the load on the heart that subclinical coronary disease has become overt. It is the surgeon's duty to exclude such a possibility before treating the patient symptomatically by means of nitrites.

13 Postoperative pulmonary complications

PULMONARY COLLAPSE

The incidence of pulmonary collapse following surgery is a function of the diagnostic criteria used and the diligence with which the condition is sought, hence the great variation in the statistics quoted for this complication of abdominal and thoracic surgery, which vary between 2.5 and 70% according to the reviewer.

However, there is little doubt that significant collapse is much more common in:

1. The presence of pre-existing pulmonary disease.
2. Following upper abdominal rather than lower abdominal incisions. This is not surprising when the difference between the effects of these incisions on the postoperative pulmonary function is considered, for after upper abdominal incisions the total lung capacity is reduced by some 2.4 litres, and by the second postoperative day the peak expiratory flow rate (PEFR) is reduced by some 50%.
3. Patients in whom peritoneal irritation is present.
4. Obese patients.
5. Cigarette smokers, in whom the bronchial secretion is increased and ciliary paralysis is common.

Even in a patient with previously healthy lungs, impairment of oxygenation of the arterial blood normally occurs for at least 48 hours following an operation, due to a reduction in the functional residual capacity. This reduction is chiefly related to the site of the operation, being greater after upper than after lower abdominal incisions. The effect is produced by an increase in gas trapping in the dependent and more richly perfused regions of the lungs.

117

The basic pathogenic mechanisms leading to pulmonary collapse include:

1. An increase in the volume of bronchial secretions due to irritation of the bronchial mucosa by the volatile anaesthetic gases. This increase is greater in patients suffering from chronic bronchitis or in heavy smokers, both of which groups are also disadvantaged by inadequate ciliary activity.
2. An increased viscosity of the secretions due to the premedication.
3. Diminished tidal volume due to postoperative pain.

The development of collapse has classically been thought to result from the formation of a mucous plug occluding either a segmental or lobar bronchus, with the result that air is resorbed distally and the affected alveoli collapse. However, it is now thought that the sequence of events is somewhat reversed.

When the lung operates at low volumes, near the residual volume, the most vulnerable portion of the air-conducting pathways are the small airways of less than 1-mm diameter. The term, 'closing volume', has been used to describe the lung volume at which closure of the small airways begins, and it is possible to measure this volume clinically. Dependent or compressed portions of the lung are the first to experience airway closure, as their regional volume is less than that of segments which are non-dependent. After the small airways close, gas is trapped distally in the alveoli and, as it is resorbed, collapse results. An important factor is the gas mixture the patient is breathing. If it is low in nitrogen and high in oxygen, the tendency of the alveoli to collapse is greater because the alveolar gas is resorbed more rapidly. This appears to be the principle reason why anaesthesia predisposes to collapse. Even in a healthy patient, collapse can occur quite rapidly. Once a segment has developed airway closure and collapsed, air movement in the bronchus to that area ceases and secretions tend to pool there, forming the mucous plug which was once thought to be the primary cause of the condition. Factors which operate to exacerbate the effects of airway closure are the volume of tracheal secretions and the ability of the patient to clear these. A further factor is loss of surfactant, which is altered by surgery, trauma, and anaesthesia and is reduced once collapse has occurred, making re-expansion of the affected segment more difficult.

Clinical presentation

Even in the absence of routine examination, attention will be drawn to the possibility of pulmonary collapse by the dramatic rise in the temperature, pulse and respiration rate which usually occurs on the second day. The greater the amount of lung tissue involved, the greater the magnitude of these changes. In addition, when massive collapse is present involving a whole lower lobe, cyanosis may be present due to the affected lung tissue acting as an arteri-ovenous shunt. Similarly, in patients previously suffering from a reduction in pulmonary function prior to the operation, a lesser degree of collapse will result in cyanosis. Clinical examination at this time may reveal diffuse as well as local signs in the lung fields, depending on whether the patient was previously suffering from pulmonary disease. The classic signs of collapse are movement of the trachea towards the side of the lesion, and diminished movement of the chest wall over the affected area. Percussion will reveal dullness over the affected area, and auscultation will show reduced, altered or absent breath sounds. Classically, bronchial breathing will be found and, in some areas, crepitations. In the presence of these signs any further investigations can be regarded as confirmatory.

Radiological diagnosis

The radiological appearances caused by 'collapse' of various parts of the lung are influenced by the presence of pre-existing disease, the relative fixity of the mediastinum and the chest wall, the presence of pleural adhesions and the presence or absence of fluid in the chest. If there is neither air nor fluid in the pleural cavity, and the lung tissue was relatively normal before collapse occurred, the same basic changes occur whichever segment or lobe is involved. Each lobe has been likened to a pyramid, the apex of which is at the hilum and the base, covered with visceral pleura, in close approximation to the parietal pleura. When a lobe becomes airless and collapses, two surfaces of the pyramid come together, but the apex remains fixed and the base always maintains conti-nuity with the parietal pleura. As a result, a flattened triangle of tissue is produced, which is seen on the plain X-ray as a shadow of increased density, possibly adjacent to an area of greater radio-translucency.

When pulmonary collapse occurs, the following changes may be seen on the plain PA and lateral films of the chest:

1. The presence of a local increase in density.
2. Displacement of the interlobar fissures. Viewed on a lateral film, the oblique fissure separating the upper and the lower lobes can normally be seen running from the level of the third thoracic spine obliquely downwards and forwards to end opposite the sixth costochondral junction. On the left there is usually no further subdivision, but on the right a horizontal fissure runs forwards from the oblique, starting in the mid-axillary line and passing forwards to the fourth costal cartilage anteriorly.

   When a lower lobe collapses, the oblique fissure swings downwards and backwards. Such displacement is usually most obvious in the lateral view, but it can also be seen in a PA projection as a density with a sharply defined upper border extending obliquely downwards and laterally from the region of the hilum. When the collapse is extensive and severe, the affected lobe moves postero-medially, occupying the posterior costophrenic gutter and the medial costovertebral angle. If the physical signs are present on the left side of the chest, it is important that the PA film is penetrating in order to show the lung shadow through the overlying cardiac shadow.

   Upper lobe collapse is usually very easily recognised. In PA projections, the horizontal fissure undergoes the most displacement but the oblique fissure also moves upwards and forwards on an axis centred upon the hilum.

In addition to these major signs, other evidence of collapse may be present, including:

3. Elevation of the diaphragm on the affected side.
4. Mediastinal shift
5. Compensatory emphysema elsewhere in the lung fields.

When the patient does not suffer the same dramatic deterioration but there is obviously increasing respiratory embarrassment, it is probable that diffuse areas of segmental collapse have occurred. This type of illness is more commonly seen in the chronic bronchitic patient, and usually develops into a bronchopneumonic condition from which the patient normally recovers following suitable treatment with physiotherapy and appropriate antibiotic therapy. In this type of patient, the plain X-ray of the chest shows patchy consolidation which may be associated with some displacement of the major fissures if the affected lung has decreased in volume.

Blood gas analysis

When any of the clinical signs already described are present, the blood gases should be measured. Although the level to which the $Pa\text{CO}_2$ rises gives some indication of the degree of respiratory failure, the accompanying effect on the acid-base balance is of greater physiological importance. Once the arterial pH falls from the normal value of 7.35–7.45 to 7.25 or below, some form of assisted ventilation is usually required. In pulmonary collapse, this is chiefly due to atrioventricular shunting but, in addition, areas of consolidation lead to lack of pulmonary compliance, increased work of respiration and, finally, fatigue of the respiratory muscles producing a diminishing respiratory effort.

Prophylaxis

There are many reports in the literature which indicate that preoperative breathing exercises reduce the incidence of collapse, especially in those patients suffering from chronic pulmonary disease associated with excessive sputum production.

Treatment of the established condition

The non-invasive treatment of pulmonary collapse is designed to increase the functional lung capacity, to increase ventilation by encouraging or, if necessary, coercing the patient to breath more deeply, and to abolish the infective element which is always associated with the condition. These end points may be achieved in the following ways:

1. *Intensive physiotherapy.* This includes both passive and active components. The former by means of postural drainage and the latter by means of percussion, vibration and assisted expiratory effort, performed by forcibly compressing the lung tissue by intermittent external pressure on the chest wall after the patient has made his maximal inspiratory effort. A further means of encouraging expansion in the conscious patient is by

intermittent positive pressure breathing (IPPB), for example using a Bird respirator.

2. *Bronchodilators.* Salbutamol can be given orally or by means of an aerosol. Administered orally in a dose of 2–4 mg three times a day the bronchodilator effect begins immediately. Alternatively, if there is a large component of bronchospasm, a slow intravenous injection of aminophylline 250–500 mg can be given dissolved in 10 ml of normal saline.

3. In order to reduce the viscosity of the sputum, a variety of medications have been used but none have proved as effective as the use of humidified air.

4. *Treatment of the associated infection.* The specific identification of the infective organism should be made if possible. Specimens of expectorated sputum are normally used for this purpose, but give somewhat inaccurate results since the expectorate is contaminated by oral organisms. To obtain an accurate specimen, a catheter is passed into the trachea and the secretions collected in a trap when suction is applied. The organisms most commonly isolated are *Streptococcus pneumoniae* and *Haemophilus influenzae*, against which the antibiotic ampicillin, 250–500 mg four times daily is active. However, other common organisms which can be isolated, especially in a hospital environment, include *Staphylococcus*, *Klebsiella*, *Pseudomonas* and a variety of Gram-negative organisms, necessitating the use of cotrimoxazole or a cephalosporin.

The resolution of the condition is marked by a dramatic improvement in the patient's general condition, the resolution of the physical signs and a return to normal of the temperature, pulse and respiratory rate. If, however, this does not occur within 24–48 hours, more active measures are required.

One of the safest and most effective manoeuvres for producing coughing is the passage of an endobronchial catheter through the nose. If the patient has copious secretions it can be connected to a suction apparatus and the secretions removed. Since this method induces a severe fit of coughing in the conscious patient as the catheter passes through the larynx into the trachea, the patient must be adequately sedated, even though this may in theory adversely affect respiration.

Such is the efficacy of the above methods, that bronchoscopy, once regarded as the primary manoeuvre in the treatment of collapse, is now rarely used. Its importance is further diminished as it is now appreciated that the 'mucous plug' once thought to be the primary cause of the condition is rarely found.

Should the patient with pre-existing lung disease develop massive collapse, respiratory failure may follow. In such a patient, the failure to eliminate CO_2 and thus carbonic acid leads to a respiratory acidosis. Thus, in the presence of tachypnoea, a P_{CO_2} in excess of 50 mmHg (6.75 kPa) and arterial hypoxaemia, there is an indication for intubation and ventilation, using machines providing positive end-expiratory pressure (PEEP) or continuous positive airway pressure (CPAP).

PULMONARY EMBOLISM

Like phlebothrombosis in the calf veins (see Chapter 14), pulmonary emboli are common following surgical procedures when no prophylactic measures have been taken. Like thrombosis in the legs, the majority cause no symptoms and pass unnoticed by both the patient and his attendants. Postmortem studies have shown that emboli rarely occur before the age of 30, but thereafter become increasingly common. By the age of 70, in nearly 60% of patients dying of causes other than a pulmonary embolus, histological evidence of embolization can be found in the branches of the pulmonary artery.

Whilst the majority of overt emboli occur between the 10th and 14th postoperative days, it is not unusual for emboli to interrupt a perfectly normal convalescence after several weeks.

Clinical presentation

The clinical presentation of a pulmonary embolus may take several forms:

1. Sudden syncope, which may be followed almost immediately by death.
2. Sudden onset of chest pain not dissimilar to that of a myocardial infarction, which may be followed by hypotension. This syndrome usually occurs when a major part of the pulmonary arterial system has been occluded so that the cardiac output suddenly diminishes. If the patient recovers, dyspnoea, tachycardia and fever rapidly follow.
3. Dyspnoea and chest pain. Dyspnoea occurs in about half of all

patients; chest pain is equally common and may be of either coronary or pleuritic type. Pleuritic pain indicates that infarction has occurred at the periphery of the lung.

4. Haemoptysis. This occurs in about one-third of all patients when blood is expectorated mixed with a little frothy sputum. Physical examination may reveal tachypnoea, dyspnoea, cyanosis and sometimes physical signs such as decreased breath sounds, rales, rhonchi and/or a pleural rub. The number and severity of the physical signs found depend in part on the position of the embolized portion of the lung and in part on the degree of arterial occlusion.

Investigation of suspected pulmonary embolus

The diagnosis of a suspected pulmonary embolus can be confirmed or refuted by a number of investigations, although the only infallible diagnosis is by pulmonary angiography.

1. Plain X-ray. The majority of pulmonary emboli produce few if any recognizable changes on a plain X-ray, because fairly large blood vessels must be occluded before changes become apparent. The changes which should be looked for include:

a. Line shadows which usually take the form of linear areas of increased density 1–3 mm thick, forming horizontal lines in the lower lobes. Serial X-rays frequently show these lines becoming more obvious with the passage of time.

b. When actual infarction has occurred, segmental shadows appear in the lung fields. These are wedged-shaped, the base being contiguous with the visceral pleural surface and with an apex which may be rounded, directed towards the hilum.

c. Other, less obvious signs on a plain X-ray may include an increase in the diameter of the pulmonary artery on the affected side, dilatation of the right ventricle and, following a large infarct from which recovery has occurred, a pleural effusion which if aspirated is bloodstained.

2. Electrocardiographic changes. These consist, when present, of the appearance of an S wave in lead I and an inverted Q wave or T wave or both in lead III.

3. Biochemical changes. Following a recent pulmonary embolus, the concentration of lactic dehydrogenase may rise well above the normal level of 90–350 IU/1.

4. Lung scan. The lungs may be scanned following the injection of macroaggregates of albumin tagged with a variety of isotopes. The macroaggregates, 2–3 times the size of red cells, block the lung capillaries but are easily fragmented and therefore produce only temporary occlusion. The final appearance of the scan is considerably influenced by the posture adopted during the procedure, because the pulmonary circulation is a low pressure system; in the erect position, the lung fields are normally increasingly dense from the apices to the bases. An even distribution of the isotope is achieved by slowly injecting the macroaggregate following a few deep breaths by the patient.

The characteristic abnormality indicating the presence of a pulmonary embolus is a segmental defect in the scan. The change is wholly non-specific, indicating merely the presence of a perfusion defect, but the probability of an embolus is increased considerably when no radiological abnormality is present on the plain X-ray. Serial scanning shows in a typical case the remarkable rapidity with which emboli can be cleared.

5. *Ventilation scanning*. This is commonly performed using Xenon 133 and will differentiate the defects due to obstructive airway disease since in all these latter conditions both the perfusion and ventilation scans are abnormal. When both the plain X-ray and ventilation scans are normal, the defects shown in the perfusion scan are presumed to be due to pulmonary embolism.

6. *Venography*. Venography is frequently performed (in the manner to be described) in patients who have suffered an overt pulmonary embolus. It permits an assessment of probable recurrence and hence can be used in some patients to indicate the necessity or otherwise of taking preventative action in the form of caval interruption. This may be either by surgery, now rarely performed, or by the insertion of a filter to prevent further emboli reaching the lungs.

7. *Pulmonary angiography*. To perform this invasive procedure, a catheter must be inserted into the pulmonary artery. This permits the injection of dye and also enables the pressure in the right ventricle and the pulmonary artery to be measured. Angiography is, however, of little use if the embolus has fragmented and so gained access to the smaller vessels. The classical sign is either a 'cut-off' or a filling defect in a segmental artery or arteries. One of the advantages of pulmonary angiography is the ease with which filling defects in the lower lobes, which are the most frequently affected, can be identified, since these are the most difficult to visualize effectively by radioisotope scanning.

Treatment

Treatment of overt embolization depends on the degree of physiological disturbance produced and on the facilities available to the surgeon. Massive pulmonary embolus is followed by death within two hours of the event in 66% of those affected, emphasizing the urgency of the condition if other than minor symptoms occur.

In a patient suffering from chest pain and/or haemoptysis, the usual treatment is immediate anticoagulation using high doses of heparin, 15 000 IU 4-hourly for 24 hours. Heparin not only has an anticoagulant effect but also, by reason of its serotonin-blocking action, reduces pulmonary vascular and bronchial vasoconstriction. The effect on the embolus itself is thought to be negligible, the chief benefit coming from the prevention of further episodes. Within 30–60 minutes of administration intravenously, the activated partial thromboplastin time (APTT) should be estimated to ensure that the required effect has been achieved. If the APTT has not reached $2-2\frac{1}{2}$ times the normal value, more heparin should be given immediately. In general, an average daily dose of 20 000–30 000 IU by continuous infusion, or 5000–10 000 units every 6 hours by intermittent injection is required. Bleeding following heparin therapy of this magnitude is unlikely to occur after the fifth postoperative day, except in patients with known platelet defects, hepatic or renal disease, septicaemia or some unassociated condition which is likely to bleed, such as an active peptic ulcer. In patients in whom severe embolization has occurred leading to 'collapse' but not immediate death, a decision must be reached as to whether to use thrombolytic agents, such as streptokinase, urokinase or recombinant tissue plasminogen activator, or perform a pulmonary embolectomy.

Evidence derived from the Urokinase Pulmonary Embolus Trial of 1973 (published in Circulation 47 Supplement 2 of that year) showed that patients receiving thrombolytic agents appeared to improve more rapidly than those given heparin alone, but no randomized trials have been performed. When using streptokinase, 250 000 units is administered intravenously over the first 30 minutes, followed by 100 000 units per hour for 48–72 hours. The thrombin clotting time should be measured before, at 12 hours and then every 24 hours after commencing therapy, the aim being values of 2–4 times the original measurement.

Pulmonary embolectomy

Patients in whom pulmonary embolectomy is indicated fall into two groups:

1. Patients so severely haemodynamically compromised that a trial of thrombolytic therapy is inappropriate.
2. Patients in whom thrombolytic therapy is contraindicated, e.g. due to recent surgery, a recent cerebrovascular accident or an active gastrointestinal lesion which is liable to bleed.

All patients in whom operation is contemplated must be investigated by means of angiography.

The first operation for this condition was described by Trendelenberg in 1908: after exposing the pulmonary artery the thrombus was removed, an operation followed by a relatively low success rate and now completely abandoned.

Subsequent technical advances have included outflow and inflow occlusion, and more recently, embolectomy has been performed using cardiopulmonary bypass and, after removing the main embolus, harvesting of the smaller fragments by balloon catheter.

If cardiac arrest has not occurred prior to this procedure, a mortality of some 10% has been reported; if cardiac arrest precedes surgery the mortality is as high as 60%.

FAT EMBOLUS

Fat embolus was first described in 1862 by Zenker, who observed the presence of fat in the lungs of a man dying from a crushing injury. In 1873, von Bergmann reported the first case in which a clinical diagnosis was made, and in 1880 Scriba described the presence of fat in the urine.

The condition is probably a common subclinical event following bony injury, but the frequency with which such emboli cause clinical disease remains unknown. In a large series of 789 trauma cases reported by Robb-Smith in 1941, there were 125 deaths, in 41 of which fat emboli were found at postmortem; of these patients death was attributed to this condition in 29 cases. During the Korean War, 39% of a group of 79 casualties dying as a result of their injuries were found to have suffered from fat emboli, and in 10 of these emboli were considered to be a major cause of death.

The generally accepted theory of causation is the simple mechanistic theory. Following a fracture, neutral fat intravasates into the circulation by a shift in the hydraulic equilibrium, to become lodged primarily in the lungs but also in the capillaries of the brain, kidneys and skin. An alternative hypothesis, the physiochemical theory, was proposed by Lehman and Moore in 1927; they considered that major trauma altered the natural emulsion of fat within the bloodstream leading to the formation of larger droplets which acted as emboli.

Clinical presentation

Typically, the respiratory and neurological signs of fat embolus appear 2–3 days after injury. The usual pulmonary symptoms are tachypnoea associated with dyspnoea, tachycardia and fever. As the condition worsens, so profuse tracheobronchial secretion develops, and fat droplets may be found in the sputum.

In severe cases, the patient becomes increasingly hypoxic and hypotensive. Occasionally, hypotension may rapidly develop due to mechanical obstruction of the pulmonary bed. If the brain is involved in a hitherto conscious patient, headache, restlessness, anxiety and deepening unconsciousness occur and, in some patients, hyperpyrexia. One of the classic signs of fat embolism is the transient appearance of petechiae in the skin of the neck, anterior chest wall, axillae and conjunctivae. As stated, fat droplets may be found in the urine or emboli in the retina. If the patient is unconscious from the outset and is being ventilated, the first indication that fat emboli are causing difficulties may be the decreasing lung compliance.

As the condition develops, so examination of the blood gases shows a fall in the Pao_2 due to a diffusion block, and radiographs of the chest show the presence of fluffy deposits similar to those seen in pulmonary oedema.

Pathology

The first indication that a biochemical process was involved came in 1940, when it was observed that patients exhibiting signs of fat embolus also had a raised serum lipase activity. Neutral fat is itself innocuous; the disastrous consequences of fat emboli result from the hydrolysis of neutral fat to fatty acids. Experimentally, these cause a disruption of the pulmonary capillary membranes, the degree of which depends on the dose administered.

The development of the syndrome caused by fat thus occurs in two phases:

1. *A mechanical phase*, as the neutral fat impacts in the various capillary beds. In the lungs, this gives rise to an immediate decrease in pulmonary compliance, an increase in perfusion pressure and an increasing load on the right heart.
2. *A chemical phase*, coming after a short interval, in which due to an increased secretion of lipase by the lung tissues, neutral fat is converted to fatty acids and glycerol. The fatty acids act locally to produce:
   a. An increase in capillary permeability, thereby causing pulmonary oedema together with destruction of the capillary walls leading to haemorrhages.
   b. Destruction of the alveolar architecture.
   c. Reduction in surfactant secretion due to destruction of the type 1 pneumocytes.

Treatment

1. The condition is self-limiting, the intravasation occurring immediately after injury. It is believed that the severity of the condition can be reduced by gentle handling of fractures, by immediate immobilization and, possibly, by early decompression of fracture haematomata. The converse – that repeated manipulation worsens the condition – is perhaps equally true.

2. In patients in whom the PaO_2 cannot be maintained at reasonable levels, oxygen by mask or by ventilation must be given (see ARDS).

3. Correction of the shock state if present.

Other treatments which have been proposed include:

4. The use of heparin. Heparin in vivo clears lipaemic plasma. However in the experimental animal, heparin fails to alleviate the condition and even increases the mortality.

5. Low molecular weight dextrans, in the hope that they might increase capillary flow and hence reduce pulmonary stagnation.

6. High doses of corticosteroids, giving 1–2 g daily. The

theoretical basis for such treatment is that by blocking the inflammatory response local blood flow will be increased, resulting in an improvement of the hypoxia, acidosis and the binding of free fatty acid by albumin. In one series reported by Fisher and his co-workers, it was claimed that corticosteroids given in large doses did indeed produce a rapid improvement in lung compliance and a return of the Pao_2 to normal within 72 hours.

ASPIRATION PNEUMONIA

In the surgical patient, aspiration of gastric contents into the respiratory tract is most commonly seen when a patient who has not starved prior to operation or who is suffering from intestinal obstruction, regurgitates at the time of anaesthetic induction before the anaesthetist has had time to inflate the cuff of the endotracheal tube. It is also seen occasionally in patients who have developed acute gastric dilatation followed by 'shock' and who, having lost their cough reflex, suddenly vomit large quantities of gastric contents.

Because the right main bronchus is more in line with the trachea than the left, aspirated material, having passed through the larynx, usually travels down the right main bronchus to reach the axillary segments of the right upper lobe and the apical segments of the right lower lobe, these being the most dependent parts when the patient is lying on the operating table.

The result of such an accident is a chemical pneumonia that is usually followed by a secondary bacterial infection; this results in necrosis of the consolidated areas and, instead of pus, a slimy fluid exudes from the necrotic areas. This is due to the fact that the organisms most commonly found are the Gram-negative *Bacteroides* and *Fusobacterium sp.*, *anaerobic cocci* and Gram-negative bacilli belonging to the *Corynebacterium* and, less commonly, the *Clostridium sp.*

Treatment

Immediately regurgitation begins, a steep head-down tilt of the operating table is required. The pharynx should be cleared by suction and, after oxygenation of the patient with a face mask, an endotracheal tube should be passed or, if already in place, the cuff should be inflated and an endobronchial catheter passed to aspirate the trachea and bronchi. This is followed by pulmonary inflation using 100% oxygen. Bronchial lavage using normal saline has been recommended by some authorities, injecting saline into the bronchi and aspirating it forthwith.

As soon as possible, an intravenous injection of hydrocortisone 500 mg should be given followed by 250 mg 4-hourly; this treatment is based on the anti-inflammatory action of the glucocorticoids and the reduction of bronchospasm which follows their administration. If bronchospasm is not controlled by this measure, a bronchodilator such as aminophyline or salbutamol should be given.

Anti-anaerobic antibiotics should be commenced immediately, after which the patient must be carefully watched in case the complications of pulmonary oedema, respiratory failure or lung abscess develop.

LUNG ABSCESS

A lung abscess is a localized area of destruction of lung parenchyma, in which infection by a pyogenic organism results in tissue necrosis and suppuration. Lung abscesses may be single or multiple and they frequently contain air-fluid levels. Small abscesses are sometimes arbitrarily described as manifestations of necrotizing or suppurative pneumonia, but they remain an expression of the same pathological process.

Lung abscesses may be preceded by any of the complications previously described in this chapter, but their overall incidence has declined due to better pre- and postoperative care and the introduction of powerful antimicrobial agents.

The commonest source of infection is the aspiration of saliva, which is rich in anaerobic bacteria even in a healthy individual and several-hundred-fold richer in the presence of dental or periodontal sepsis. Small amounts of saliva are normally aspirated during sleep in many normal individuals, and in an even greater number of patients subjected to anaesthesia and sedation. The commonest sites of abscess formation are the apical segments of the lower lobes or the posterior segments of the upper lobes as those are the most dependent parts of the lung when the patient is lying on his back or side. The organisms most commonly present in an established abscess are the anaerobic *Bacteroides sp.* especially *Bacteroides melaninogenicus* and the aerobic *Klebsiella pneumoniae* and *Pseudomonas aeruginosa*.

Presentation

The commonest mode of presentation in the postoperative surgical patient is the failure of recovery from one of the pulmonary complications previously described in this chapter. Fever, instead of resolving continues, frequently associated with chills, rigors, purulent sputum, increasing dyspnoea and chest pain. Since the majority of abscesses rupture into a bronchus rather than the pleural cavity at some point, large quantities of purulent sputum may be expectorated, with the putrid smell indicative of an anaerobic infection.

On clinical examination of the chest there are no physical signs which are specific to a lung abscess. Signs of consolidation or a friction rub may be present. In the past, the so-called 'cavernous' breath sounds associated with large cavities were described and regarded as pathognomonic of the condition. Should the abscess rupture into the pleural cavity – a rare event – signs of a pleural effusion or empyema may be found.

Radiology

Early in the course of their development, abscesses merely appear as segmental shadows with the border blurred and slightly irregular because of oedema in adjacent segments. Once the abscess has ruptured into a bronchus, it appears as a translucent ring containing a fluid level in the middle of the opaque segment. Occasionally, a lung slough is seen as a rounded or oval opacity within the cavity which usually liquefies and disappears within 1–2 weeks; this distinguishes it from a mycetoma, in which the slough is permanent. A pleural effusion may also be present if the inflammatory process has involved the pleura.

Treatment

The treatment of lung abscess is essentially conservative and following the administration of appropriate antibiotics it is now unusual for operative intervention to be necessary. In one reported series, 70% of the cavities disappeared within three months. A suitable antibiotic regime consists of metronidazole, 500 mg 8-hourly by infusion, together with benzlpenicillin, 5–10 mu per day intravenously. The latter drug is used because some of the anaerobic cocci and most microphillic streptococci are resistant to metronidazole. In addition to antibiotics, physiotherapy including postural drainage and percussion is required to clear the lung of purulent material. The duration of treatment is determined by the response, but it may be necessary to continue with the above measures for several months in order to achieve a cure and prevent relapse.

In only a very small number of cases is surgical intervention required, but if closed drainage – the first step – fails, lobectomy may be required.

ADULT RESPIRATORY DISTRESS SYNDROME

The adult respiratory distress syndrome (ARDS) – originally known as 'shock lung' or 'post-traumatic wet lung' – was first recognized some thirty years ago when it was observed that some patients suffering from septicaemia, severe trauma, pancreatitis or receiving a massive blood transfusion developed pulmonary failure.

The condition is not uncommon. A recent survey in the United Kingdom indicated that 10–15 000 cases of the condition occurred per annum, and in the United States a survey in 1972 of over 6000 trauma cases showed that 6% developed this syndrome.

Conditions which may precipitate ARDS include tissue injury combined with shock, sepsis, burns in which smoke inhalation has occurred, aspiration and lung contusions. In many series, the overall mortality is of the order of 60% and if the condition follows septic shock mortality rates can reach as high as 90%.

Clinical presentation

Typically the condition presents 48–72 hours after the initial insult, at which time the individual may even appear to be improving. In the conscious patient who is not on a ventilator, increasing restlessness, tachycardia and tachypnoea develop.

If the patient is already being ventilated, a rapid reduction in lung compliance is noted. At this point, a chest X-rays shows widespread bilateral infiltrates which, over the next several hours, spread to become confluent as extensive alveolar oedema and haemorrhage develop, although the apices may be spared. Measurement of respiratory function, in addition to revealing diminishing compliance, also reveals a reduction in functional lung capacity, an increasing ventilation/perfusion mismatch and increasing pulmonary shunting as the condition progresses.

Analysis of the blood gases indicates both a reduced Po_2 and Pco_2, although in the later stages as the physiological dead space increases, so the Pco_2 rises.

Once the syndrome is initiated it is irreversible, death occurring within seven days from respiratory failure or later from broncho-pneumonia. In those patients who survive, chronic respiratory problems frequently follow which are totally irreversible and may require lung transplantation.

Pathology

In the experimental animal, a similar condition can be produced by the intravenous injection of Gram-negative bacteria or endotoxin. Such treatment will produce a transient pulmonary hypertension followed by progressive lung damage commencing with pulmonary oedema, itself caused by increased capillary permeability. This experimental work gave rise to the concept that low-pressure (permeability) oedema was the central initiating event in ARDS and that all other pathological changes were secondary. The secondary changes, including haemorrhage and the development of thrombi, occurred (so it was thought) when the interstitial oedema damaged the alveolar walls, and atelectasis developed because of diminished surfactant. However, it is now considered that complement-induced neutrophil aggregation in the lung capillaries is the important feature of the disease, a concept supported by the correlation which exists between the onset of the syndrome, its severity and the circulating levels of complement C5.

The importance of the neutrophils is also supported by experimental work showing that the syndrome is limited if neutropenia is first induced prior to 'triggering' the syndrome.

After the initial aggregation of the neutrophils, the capillary damage is now thought to result from free radicals of O_2 generated by the activated white cells. This hypothesis is supported by the finding that the hydrogen peroxide level in the expired air of patients on mechanical respiration who are developing ARDS rises in comparison with those patients who do not develop the syndrome. A further finding supporting the importance of the neutrophil is a rise in the plasma lysozyme which is a measure of the in vivo turnover of neutrophils.

Recently, interest has passed to the possible role of the eicosanoids. Various metabolites of arachidonic acid can mimic virtually the whole range of primary and secondary pathological changes seen in ARDS; furthermore, the release of eicosanoids, often in a specific sequence, has been observed in both the human syndrome and in animal models. In the experimental animal, drugs which inhibit the various phases of arachidonic acid metabolism can block the experimental syndrome, suggesting that at least some of the eicosanoids play an integral, rather than incidental, role in this syndrome.

Whatever the underlying cause of ARDS, the pathological features remain constant. In the alveoli, interstitial haemorrhage and a massive infiltration with neutrophils develops. The type I alveolar cells which normally excrete surfactant and which cannot themselves proliferate are destroyed to be replaced by type II pneumocytes, some of which undergo transdifferentiation into type I cells, should the patient survive. Gross flooding of the interstitial space and the alveoli occurs with fluid so rich in plasma proteins that subsequent osmotic resorption is limited. The plasminogen system is overwhelmed, thereby allowing the deposition of a fibrin network which subsequently becomes fibrous and occludes the lymphatics.

Treatment

Several methods of treatment have been proposed, although none have yet been shown to alter the course of the disease or the prognosis. Whilst steroids should in theory have a part to play, they do not appear to be of any practical value. In experimental sheep, a combination of steroid plus a non-steroidal anti-inflammatory agent, meclofenamate sodium, has been shown virtually to abolish the response, and in humans indomethacin has been used. Experimentally, two other possible lines of therapy have been explored: the use of free radical scavengers such as N-acetyl cysteine in an attempt to limit the damage by free radicals from the aggregated neutrophils; and the administration of vitamin E, since it has been found that a significant reduction in the level of this vitamin occurs as the disease progresses.

In practical terms, however, the established treatment consists of:

1. The control of sepsis if this is present.

2. The rigid control of fluid balance in order to limit the increasing pulmonary oedema.
3. The correction of the hypoxaemia.

This last may be achieved by the simple use of one of a variety of a face masks, such as the Hudson or the Venturi, both of which can provide concentrations of oxygen in the region of 60%.

If the patient is intolerant of a mask, nasal spectacles can be used which provide oxygen at a concentration of between 20–45%. All oxygen-enriched air should be humidified by passage through a humidifier.

When the situation is more serious, and the patient is deteriorating with the Po_2 falling below 60 mmHg (8.0 kPa), one of two alternative methods of ventilation may assist survival:

Intermittent positive pressure ventilation (IPPV). This may improve matters by reducing the ventilation/perfusion imbalance as a result of:

1. Recruiting previously closed alveoli by providing the necessary opening pressure.
2. Improving the distribution of gases in the lungs.

In addition, the work of breathing is decreased.

Pulmonary end expiratory pressure (PEEP). This method may improve matters by:

1. Increasing the functional residual capacity.
2. Improving the ventilation/perfusion ratio.
3. Increasing the Po_2 for a given concentration of inspired oxygen.

14 Other postoperative complications

DEEP VENOUS THROMBOSIS

Assuming that no prophylactic action is taken, it has now been established that some 30% of all surgical patients develop a deep venous thrombosis, although the incidence varies somewhat according to the type of operation. Thus, major abdominal operations are followed by a 30% risk, the incidence rising to 50% following orthopaedic operations, particularly those associated with the hip and lower limbs. Factors increasing the risk of phlebothrombosis include:

1. Cardiac disease.
2. Increasing age.
3. Obesity.
4. Anaemia.
5. Polycythaemia.
6. Debility.
7. Hemiplegia.
8. Malignant disease.
9. Splenectomy.
10. Contraceptive pills containing a high oestrogen content.

In the past, the occurrence of postoperative thrombosis in the deep veins of the lower limb was diagnosed entirely on clinical grounds, but it eventually became evident that in the majority of individuals dying from massive pulmonary embolization, no antecedent diagnosis of phlebothrombosis had been made. Clinically, the earliest physical sign which may draw attention to a developing phlebothrombosis is a rise in the pulse rate, but this can usually only be detected if a 4-hourly chart is being used to record this parameter; it is, in any case, often so transient that it can easily be missed. Later, perhaps, and classically on or about the fifth postoperative day, the patient may be aware of a pain in the calf, particularly on getting out of bed, although many patients will dismiss this, thinking of it merely as a cramp following prolonged recumbency and lack of exercise. Should the thrombus extend from the calf, some swelling of the leg may develop, if even greater extension occurs to the ilio-femoral segment, this leads to the classic condition of phlegmasia alba dolens (the white leg) or to the more serious condition of phlegmasia caerulea dolens – the blue or purple leg, in which there is a danger that some loss of superficial tissues of the toes may occur.

It has now been established that extension of the thrombus from the leg veins of the calf to the popliteal vein greatly increases the risk of pulmonary embolization. Fortunately, whilst calf vein thrombosis is common, extension above the knee is comparatively rare. Out of a collected series of 4000 intensively investigated patients to whom no prophylactic treatment had been given, such extenson occurred in only 6.4%. However, it follows that if prophylactic measures are to be taken, they should begin before the thrombotic process has begun or certainly whilst it is still limited to the calf. The period of greatest danger is immediately after an operation and during the first two postoperative days. During this period, a deficiency of plasminogen activator causes a reduction of the blood fibrinolytic activity, in addition to other factors, including stasis and, possibly, changes in the vessel walls; these three precipitating factors constituting Virchow's triad.

Detection

In the recent past, efforts have been made to determine the onset and the extent of the thrombus. One method of determining the presence of a calf vein thrombosis is the detection of radioactivity in a thrombus or clot which is incorporating within its structure isotopically labelled fibrinogen. The principles of this method were first described by Hobbs and Davies in 1960, and later adapted for use in humans in 1965 by Atkins and Hawkins, who found using this test that the number of false-positives was as low as 2%.

One method of performing this type of test is as follows. The thyroid uptake of the isotope is first blocked by the daily administration of 150 mg of sodium iodide, commencing with a first dose 24 hours prior to beginning the investigation and continuing for some 28 days thereafter. Each limb is then marked at 15-cm intervals from above and below the knee joint, and at the completion of the operation 100 µCi of ^{125}I-labelled fibrinogen is administered intravenously. A daily count is then made over each mark using a portable ratemeter, the count being expressed as a percentage of the radioactivity detected over the praecordium. The line of the count should extend from the midpoint of the inguinal ligament to the adductor tubercle, and then from the centre of the popliteal fossa to the ankle. Counts are performed with the legs elevated to 30° above the horizontal. When expressed as a percentage of the praecordial count, the count at the inguinal ligament is normally about 56, and at the midcalf, 25, the count slowly decreasing towards the ankle.

The presence of thrombus or clot is indicated by a rise in the count over a certain point in the limb, the so-called 'hot spot'. To be meaningful, it must cause a rise in the count of 15% or more, and it should persist and even increase in both magnitude and extent on succeeding days.

Most investigators consider this test capable of diagnosing thrombus formation in about 90% of those affected from a point some 10 cm inferior to the inguinal ligament and below, but consider it useless for the diagnosis of thrombosis in the common femoral and iliac veins. It is, of course, obvious that the presence of a haematoma in either leg completely invalidates this method, and it is therefore useless following arterial surgery.

Although the method is effective, it has two disadvantages: firstly, an available isotope source is required, and secondly, it is somewhat time-consuming and relatively boring to perform. It cannot therefore be accepted as a routine clinical investigation, and its use must be restricted to those at special risk.

This type of work has led to some doubt as to whether the initial starting point for the thrombotic process is always in the calf. Some believe that thrombosis may begin in the thigh and that many thrombi have a multi-centric origin, findings which tend to lessen the importance of those methods of protection, which are directed solely at diminishing calf stasis during operation by physical means.

Other diagnostic methods now available include:

1. Doppler scanning. The use of ultrasound for the detection of vessel patency and flow patterns was first described by Watson and Rushmore in 1963, and was applied to the problems associated with deep vein thrombosis in 1967 by Strandness and his colleagues, using a machine with a transmission frequency of 5 MHz. This was changed to 2MHz by Evans, in 1970, who considered the lower frequency to be more sensitive. Over a normal patent femoral vein, a sound is heard like a wind storm, cyclic in character and in phase with respiration; during inspiration the signal decreases in both amplitude and pitch and usually completely disappears at the height of inspiration. If the femoral vein is blocked by thrombus, the sound disappears altogether. This method is of little use in detecting calf vein thrombosis, but is accurate and correlates well with other methods when clotting has occurred proximal to the popliteal vein. It also has the advantage of been non-invasive and quick to perform.

2. Venography. The most accurate investigation of all is venography, a method developed by Bauer in 1940. This will demonstrate the position, size and number of thrombi, and whether the clot is loose or adherent. However, it is invasive, expensive and requires the use of relatively complex equipment. The investigation is normally carried out by injecting a radio-opaque material into a dorsal vein on the foot following the application of tourniquets or inflatable cuffs both above the ankle and above the knee at a pressure just sufficient to occlude the superficial veins. The tourniquets are essential in order to direct the flow of dye through to the deep system. If filling of the iliac and lower part of the inferior vena cava is inadequate, the injection is repeated during a violent Valsalva manoeuvre. Alternatively, the pelvic veins can be demonstrated by a pertrochanteric injection. The presence of thrombus or clot is shown by observing well-defined filling defects in the venous channels on both screening and serial films. Loose clot appears as a cylindrical or rounded translucent defect separated from the vein wall by a fine white line of contrast medium. When this line is absent, it indicates adherence of the clot, a process which is usually complete within 4 days of the clot forming.

Prophylaxis

No investigator doubts that venous thrombosis is the precursor of pulmonary emboli, which result in a mortality varying between 1 and 3% according to the series examined. For this reason, extensive therapeutic trials of a variety of measures have been undertaken in an attempt to reduce the incidence of phlebothrombosis.

These include:

1. *Intermittent pneumatic compression of the calf*, aimed at increasing the bloodflow through the lower limbs throughout operation and beyond. A typical regime is calf compression for 10 seconds per minute at an inflation pressure of 35–45 mmHg.

2. The insertion of Greenfeld filters into the inferior cava, to prevent emboli reaching the pulmonary artery. This method is invasive and therefore has a limited application. It is usually used only in patients at high risk, in patients who have already suffered a pulmonary embolus, or in patients in whom therapeutic antico-agualtion is contraindicated.

3. The use of graduated pressure elastic stockings. One of the commonly used stockings is the TED stocking which is so knitted as to stretch in one direction only, be contoured to the limb, seamless and with a gusset at the top to avoid a 'gartering' effect. Wearing the correct stocking size, the pressure at various levels of the lower limb are as follows: at the ankle, 18 mmHg; midcalf, 14 mmHg; popliteal fossa, 8 mmHg; lower thigh, 10 mmHg; and in the upper thigh, 8 mmHg. Wearing such a stocking, increased flow occurs in the lower limb, contrast medium being cleared in one-half the time of an unstockinged leg; this increase in linear flow reduces pooling in the soleal plexuses and behind the valve cusps.

4. General measures to reduce the coagulability of the blood during and after operation. Among the measures used are:

a. Dextran 70 infused during the course of the operation and for 1–7 days thereafter. Dextran acts by inhibiting the intravascular aggregation of red blood cells (sludging) and by reducing platelet aggregation.

b. Heparin which acts by enhancing the effect of antithrombin III, an α_2-globulin. Heparin together with antithrombin III inhibits the activity of activated factor X, thus inhibiting the conversion of fibrinogen to fibrin. Classified as a direct anticoagulant, it inhibits clotting both in vitro and in vivo. Heparin is a heterogenous group of polysaccharides with a molecular weight of 30 000 daltons. Recently, another product, Enoxaprin, has been produced, which is a low-molecular-weight heparin with a molecular weight of 4000–6500 daltons. More recently still, heparin with 0.5 mg of dihydroergotamine had been introduced under the name of HDHE. Dihydroergotamine is added because this drug is a vasoconstrictor which has been reported to reduce venous stasis by inducing venous constriction of the capacitant vessels of the limb.

c. Ancrod, an active enzyme principle derived from the venom of the Malayan pit viper. It acts by reducing the concentration of fibrinogen by cleavage of the microparticles which are rapidly removed from the circulation by fibrinolysis.
d. Aspirin, which is an antiplatelet agent.
e. Dipyridamole which acts by modifying platelet aggregation, adhesion and survival. Combinations of aspirin and dipyridamole have also been used.

Of these various measures, the use of heparin has received the most extensive investigation. The following regimes, using calcium heparin or heparin sodium have been proposed.

1. 5000 IU subcutaneously two hours before surgery, again 24 hours after surgery, and then every 12 hours for five days.
2. 5000 IU prior to operation and then every 12 hours for five days.
3. 200 IU/kg bodyweight for three days before operation.
4. 5000 IU two hours prior to operation and then two doses at 12-hourly intervals.
5. 5000 IU 12-hourly for five days, starting two hours before operation.
6. 10 000 IU the night prior to operation and then again 24 hours after surgery, continuing thereafter at 12-hourly intervals for five days.

In 1988, Clagett and Reisch performed an analysis of the efficacy of the different prophylactic measures which had been used for the prevention of phlebothrombosis.

Typical of their findings was the following: The data on 8000 patients was collected from a number of trials in which patients had been randomized into two groups, an untreated group and a group of equal number who had received 5000 IV of heparin two hours before operation and every 8–12 hours following surgery for seven days. The incidence of deep vein thrombosis confirmed by firbrinogen-uptake studies in the treated group was 8.7%, as compared with 25% in the controls. In 8 trials examined, the findings of the fibrinogen-uptake study were further tested by means of phlebography, when the overall incidence of deep vein thrombosis was found to be 6% in the treated group as compared to 15.4% in the controls.

Considering the more dangerous situation of extension or the presence of thrombus above the knee, the incidence was only 1.4%

in the patients receiving heparin as compared to 6.4% in the controls.

As regards the incidence of pulmonary embolus itself, only 0.5% of the treated group suffered this complication as compared to 1.2% in the controls. More important still, the incidence of fatal pulmonary embolus fell to 0.2% in those patients receiving heparin, as compared to 0.7% in the controls.

Clagett and Reisch also compared dextran with low dose heparin, and found that the latter appeared somewhat superior to dextran in preventing calf vein thrombosis. However no difference could be found when the two groups were assessed for the incidence of above knee thrombosis, neither was there a significant difference between the two groups in relation to the frequency of fatal pulmonary emboli.

With regard to the mechanical methods of prophylaxis, both intermittent pneumatic compression of the calf and graded elastic stockings appeared to be effective in reducing the incidence of calf vein thrombosis, as assessed by fibrinogen-uptake studies. In neither method was sufficient data available to assess their efficacy in preventing above knee thrombosis or their effect on the incidence of fatal pulmonary embolus.

Heparin-dihydroergotamine, the more recent combination, appeared to be marginally better than low dose heparin in preventing deep vein thrombosis but appeared to have no advantage over heparin alone in lowering the incidence of pulmonary embolus.

It is therefore proven beyond doubt that both physical and medical means can dramatically reduce the incidence of deep vein thrombosis. Using either low-dose heparin or dextran it has also become apparent that the incidence of thrombosis above the knee, pulmonary embolus itself and, most important of all, the incidence of fatal pulmonary embolus can be reduced.

Nevertheless, the price paid for this protection may be a more difficult operation, particularly when using regimes administered immediately prior to operation because of increased oozing. Furthermore, there is undoubtedly an increase in the number of wound haematomata which develop following both forms of therapy, more so after low-dose heparin. This may in turn lead to an increased rate of wound infection or deep infection around an implanted prosthesis, since blood is an ideal breeding ground for many bacteria, although this has not been statistically proven. Experimental evidence also shows that the rate of collagen synthesis is diminished by heparin, thus possibly increasing the incidence of wound dehiscence.

It is for these reasons that the use of heparin and dextran following all operations has not been adopted as routine. Their use is reserved for those patients in whom risk factors are already present prior to surgery, factors which include (apart from those already listed) a previous history of thromboembolic disease, chronic venous stasis in the lower limb or prolonged immobilization prior to surgery.

If prophylactic therapy has not been used or if, despite its usage, clinical evidence supported by phlebography confirms that a deep vein thrombosis has occurred, a heparin regime controlled by measurements of the prothrombin time should be commenced. One commonly used regime consists of the administration of 10 000 units of heparin four-hourly for 24 hours, then six-hourly. Alternatively, continuous intravenous administration can be used giving 40 000 units in the first 24 hours and thereafter 20 000 units daily. If undesirable bleeding occurs it can be treated by protamine sulphate, injecting 1 mg intravenously for every 100 units of heparin last administered.

Since anticoagulant therapy is normally continued for several weeks, particularly if thrombosis has been associated with embolism, it is customary to commence the administration of an indirect anticoagulant after 48 hours. One such drug in common use is warfarin, administering an oral dose of 50 mg followed by a continuation dose of 5–10 mg daily depending on the prothrombin time, which returns to normal within 4–5 days of ceasing its administration.

There is no well-documented account as to how long anticoagulant therapy should continue, particularly following a major thrombus or a pulmonary embolus, but as a rule of thumb a period of three months should probably elapse before ceasing treatment. This allows time for the clot to become organized, recanalized and perhaps, more importantly, re-covered by endothelium, so that reactivation of the clotting mechanism can no longer occur.

An alternative to anticoagulants is the use of streptokinase, which is a protein obtained from the culture of the haemolytic streptococcus, Lancefield Type C. This enzyme activates plasminogen to plasmin and chiefly affects thrombi which are mainly fibrinoid in character; its effect on platelet-rich white thrombi is much less evident. The side-effects of streptokinase are allergic reactions, haemorrhage and fever. Severe haemorrhage may require the administration of aminocaproic acid, giving 4–6 g immediately, followed by 1 g hourly but not exceeding 30 g in all. Fever can be controlled by corticosteroids. High antibody titres to streptokinase develop after 7–10 days or after streptococcal throat infections. Used for the treatment of massive phlebothrombosis, one suggested regime is 600 000 units infused over 30 minutes preceded by either 90 or 120 mg of plasminogen in saline infused over 4–6 hours; this regime is continued daily for 5 days.

CARDIAC ARREST AND RESUSCITATION

A cardiac arrest may occur at any time in any part of the hospital. Although 'first aid' is essential for saving life, it can only be carried out correctly if all grades of nursing and medical staff have been properly trained. Once first aid treatment has been given, skilled assistance is usually required to continue treatment successfully; therefore in every hospital some method must be devised whereby rapid communication can be established with such assistants.

Although a single individual may be able to prevent death in some cases of cardiac arrest by the immediate application of cardiopulmonary resuscitation, it requires an experienced team to continue treatment beyond the initial stages. Furthermore, unless an individual has had experience in the fields of cardiac surgery or anaesthesia, his familiarity in dealing with this condition will be extremely limited. For this reason, only the preliminary steps of cardiac resuscitation will be described, since the handling of the complex arrhythmias which may develop following restoration of the heartbeat requires more expertise and experience than is available to a single individual.

The estimated frequency of cardiac arrest, other than provocation for the purposes of open heart surgery, had been variously estimated at between 1 in 1000 and 1 in 4000 operations. The cause is usually multifactorial, the various factors involved including the anaesthetic itself, a mishap at intubation, regurgitation and vomiting, underventilation and anoxia and postoperative respiratory obstruction. Any acute episode, such as hypoxia, haemorrhage or emotion, may bring about the sudden cessation of rhythmical myocardial contractility if the heart has been damaged by ischaemia, or if the threshold for ventricular fibrillation has been lowered by the overadministration of digitalis or by valvular heart disease.

If cardiac arrest occurs, death is imminent. Within 3–4 minutes the cerebrum is damaged beyond repair, although other parts of the central nervous system have longer survival times. The cerebellum can survive for between 5 and 10 minutes, and the brainstem for 20–23 minutes.

Although the brain is only 2% of the total bodyweight, it receives 15% of the cardiac output and 20% of the oxygen uptake. Under normal circumstances, cerebral bloodflow is governed by a self-regulatory mechanism which adjusts the blood flow to need, the mechanism being governed largely by the $PaCO_2$ and the pH of the smooth muscle of the arterial wall.

The usual energy requirements of the brain are supplied from glucose and, because the brain has only a very limited capacity for anaerobic metabolism, it can incur only a limited oxygen debt. Once cardiac arrest occurs, the supply of oxygen and glucose is abolished and anaerobic metabolism begins, with the progressive accumulation of lactic and pyruvic acid. As the situation develops, cerebral function is depressed, a process which begins when the cerebral bloodflow is reduced to below 50% of its normal resting value, but permanent brain damage only occurs when the blood flow is less than 15%. Under normal circumstances, the cerebral blood flow only decreases significantly when the mean arterial pressure is below 50 mmHg or, put another way, when the cardiac output is reduced by 40% or approximately 2 l/min.

These findings explain why, when a cardiac arrest occurs, the first response must be to commence cardiac massage in an attempt to restore some degree of cerebral circulation. The initial seconds are critical. In a large survey of 177 patients, Pederson and his colleagues found that 20% of patients survived if cardiac massage was started immediately, and that for each minute of delay the mortality increased by 50%. Within the first 30 seconds, the accompanying apnoea is unimportant because the lungs normally contain sufficient oxygen to prevent harmful desaturation within this period; however within this period thought followed by action must be given to this facet of the problem.

Clinical presentation

The presenting signs of cardiac arrest, indicating an urgent need for cardiopulmonary resuscitation, obviously differ between the conscious and the unconscious or anaesthetized patient.

In the conscious patient, an abrupt loss of consciousness followed by gasping respiration with an associated absence of cardiac or major arterial pulses are important clinical criteria. As the condition develops, the pupils dilate and the skin becomes ashen grey.

In the unconscious or anaesthesized patient, the absence of a carotid pulse or, if the patient is connected to an electrocardiograph, the development of ventricular flutter, fibrillation or standstill, are all evidence that cardiac arrest has occurred. If the patient is anaesthetized, the pupillary signs may not be of great significance because of the use of opiates prior to the operation or because of the normal effects of an anaesthetic. However if the patient has received no drugs before the arrest occurs, dilatation of the pupils suggests that the arrest is of not less than 40 seconds duration.

External cardiac massage

If the chest is unopened, the diagnosis of cardiac arrest must be followed by external cardiac massage. This was first described as early as 1883 by Koenig, and was revived in the early 1950s having in the interim been superceded by internal massage. It is, however, an unacceptable technique in a patient in whom:

1. The chest is already opened.
2. A severe fixed chest deformity is present since a sternal movement of between 5 and 8 cm is required to produce adequate ventricular compression.
3. A severe chest injury has occurred, because in these circumstances the heart may be damaged by fractured ribs.
4. The heart has been displaced by a pneumothorax.
5. Cardiac tamponade is already present.

The method of manual external cardiac massage is now fairly standardized. If possible, a board or tray should be placed under the thorax with the minimum of delay. The compression force should be delivered with the heel of the hand; the hand is hyperextended at the wrist and extended at the elbow, the left hand normally overlying the right in a right-hand-dominant person. The thrust is delivered not by movements of the arm and forearm but by the bodyweight. The aim is to compress the heart between the sternum in front and the spine behind. In order to achieve this, the compression should be applied at the junction of the upper two-thirds of the sternum with the lower one-third. In infants and young children, the heart lies slightly higher and the point of maximum compression should, therefore, be the mid-sternum. If the compression force is applied elsewhere it loses its effectiveness; if it is too low and to the right, damage to the liver may occur; if too low and to the left, rupture of the stomach or regurgitation of the stomach contents may occur or the spleen be damaged. If compression is applied too vigorously, either costochondral dislocation or, more seriously, fractures of the ribs themselves may result.

The absolute effectiveness of external cardiac massage in man has been measured and compared to the effectiveness of internal massage. Expressed in terms of the cardiac index – i.e. the cardiac output in l/min per m^2 of body surface – internal massage is twice as effective as external and, in addition, produces a larger stroke index and a greater fall in the mean circulation time. However, in either method, even using 100% oxygen, the arterial Po_2 remains low due to extensive pulmonary arteriovenous shunting. It has been estimated that the critical cardiac index is approximately 2 l/min. This cannot be achieved by external massage, but can be just exceeded by internal massage.

Artificial respiration

As the seconds pass, the need to commence artificial respiration becomes more urgent. For this, a team effort is required. The methods available are discussed below.

1. Expired air resuscitation: mouth-to-mouth or mouth-to-nose

The patient's head is extended and the lower jaw brought forwards so as to lift the tongue away from the posterior pharyngeal wall. The mouth is then inspected, and dentures if present are removed as also is any obvious debris. The nose is then pinched closed, and the resuscitator takes several deep breaths and then exhales slowly into the patient's open mouth. When the chest is inflated, the resuscitator removes his mouth to allow passive expiration. If the operator hyperventilates between each attempt, his or her expired air contains only about 2% less oxygen than the ambient air. In a normal person with no deterioration of lung function, this is sufficient to prevent significant hypoxia but, unfortunately, the patient suffering from a cardiac arrest has a grossly abnormal lung function, chiefly due to arteriovenous shunting.

If mouth-to-mouth respiration is found unsatisfactory, the

mouth to nose technique can be used. This is in many ways easier and more effective, in that the mouth of the operator will almost certainly make an airtight junction around the nose of the patient.

The recommended rate of inflation is 12–16/min, and obviously the smaller the number of inflations the greater must be the volume of each. However, this may be difficult to achieve if the chest wall is already fixed as in the emphysematous patient, or if pulmonary oedema is present.

2. Bag/valve/mask system

If this equipment is available a simple airway is inserted. The oxygen is turned on to deliver 8 l/min and the mask is applied to the face. The bag is usually filled because the face is held firmly against the mask, and once filled it is squeezed firmly; a watch is made to see that the chest expands, after which the chest is allowed to deflate spontaneously.

3. Respiration through a cuffed endotracheal tube

This is the most effective way of achieving artificial ventilation. If arrest has occurred in theatre, the tube may already be in place; if not, it can be introduced. If it is impossible to open the jaws, a short-acting muscle relaxant such as suxamethonium chloride may be needed; 30 mg injected intravenously will act within 30 seconds.

Internal cardiac massage

If the heart has already been exposed by the transternal route, no further discussion is necessary. However, if the chest is unopened the question arises as to whether, despite its greater efficacy, this method should be used – the reason being the severe damage which can be done to the myocardium by too-vigorous pummelling of the flaccid muscle.

If it is decided to use this method, the most commonly used exposure is to enter the chest cavity through the fourth or fifth left intercostal space, i.e. just below the nipple line in the male or the lower attachment of the breast in the female. The incision should start 2.5 cm lateral to the margin of the sternum, so avoiding the internal mammary artery and vein, and it should be extended as far lateral as possible. When the incision is completed, a self-retaining retractor is put in place and the hand inserted into the thoracic cavity. The heart is either compressed against the back of the sternum with the flat of the right hand; or the right hand is inserted behind the heart, the left is placed in front and the heart compressed between the two. Both ventricles must be compressed and a rapid compression must be followed by a fairly prolonged interval of diastole to allow cardiac filling to occur.

Whichever method of cardiac compression is used, spontaneous cardiac activity is urgently required, because the longer the relatively ineffectual massage is continued the greater becomes the degree of metabolic acidosis. An attempt should be made to correct the acidosis by the administration of bicarbonate. The quantity of bicarbonate necessary can be estimated from the following simple formula:

$$\text{Base deficit} = \frac{\text{wt. of patient in kg}}{5} \times \text{duration of arrest in minutes} \times 0.5$$

Thus, a 70-kg male in whom a cardiac arrest has been present for 9 minutes requires an immediate injection of 65 mmol of sodium bicarbonate.

Following the correction of the acidosis, cardiac stimulants such as adrenaline can be given.

Even if spontaneous myocardial contraction is restored, this may be wholly ineffectual because of an associated dysrhythmia, the commonest of which is ventricular fibrillation.

Treatment of fibrillation

The treatment of fibrillation is to defibrillate the heart by passing a shock wave through the myocardium. The aim is to produce an instantaneous depolarization of the active cardiac muscle mass, thereby momentarily producing complete cardiac standstill. If the heart was normal before fibrillation, the sino-atrial node then resumes control and sinus rhythm develops.

All defibrillators are potentially dangerous and should therefore be handled with caution. If electrodes are held by separate operators there is no need to wear rubber gloves, but these should be worn if the resuscitator is holding both electrodes at the same time.

Electrode cream is applied to the whole of the contact surface to ensure good electrical contact and minimal skin resistance. The normal energy setting for an adult might be as high as 300 J or for a child 150 J, but these levels should not be exceeded. If the patient is known to be fully digitalized, a lower setting should be used and increased if found ineffective.

The position of the electrodes on the body is fairly critical, since an electric current passes in a straight line from electrode to electrode. One electrode should be applied to the right of the sternum and below the clavicle, and the other to the left midaxillary line at about the fifth interspace. In the chest is open, the electrode pads are soaked in normal saline and are placed on either side of the heart. This is the position of choice if the sternum has been split, but if the approach has been made under emergency conditions and the heart can only be approached from the side, the electrodes are placed in the anteroposterior axis. Following the first shock, the electrodes are left in place until the ECG reappears on the oscillograph. This normally takes one or two seconds. If the shock has had the desired effect, normal sinus rhythm will be seen to develop. However, many factors mitigate against the return of a normal rhythm, among the most important of which are the presence of a metabolic acidosis, the state of the myocardium and the duration of the fibrillation before attempting to correct it.

Since other dysrhythmias may replace simple fibrillation, it is sometimes necessary to reduce the level of myocardial irritability. Because such an action may result in complete loss of myocardial excitability, this should only be done if the resuscitator has complete confidence in the electrocardiographic diagnosis. The two commonly used drugs for this purpose are lignocaine 1 mg/kg bodyweight, and procainamide up to 1 mg by slow intravenous injection. The latter drug depresses not only myocardial irritability but also contractility so that hypotension may develop.

When fibrillation continues for more than one hour, regardless of the current used, the number of shocks and the correction of acidosis, it must be accepted that resuscitation has failed.

RENAL FAILURE

Definitions

In absolute terms, renal failure may be defined as a situation in which the volume of urine excreted by an adult falls below the level required to control the internal environment, i.e. 400–600 ml daily in a normal adult.

It is, however, more appropriate to consider renal failure in physiological terms, regarding it as a condition in which the volume of urine excreted is insufficient to prevent nitrogenous end products accumulating in the blood. This definition recognizes that, in order to maintain homeostasis, kidneys damaged by ageing, hypertension or other disease need to excrete larger volumes of urine than those commonly accepted as normal.

Aetiology

The commonest cause of renal failure in a surgical patient is hypovolaemia followed by hypotension. This situation results in prerenal failure which may progress to intrarenal failure.

The causes of hypovolaemic include:

1. Blood loss as a result of accidental or surgical trauma.
2. Plasma loss from extensive burns or severe pancreatitis.
3. Fluid and electrolyte loss following intestinal obstruction, external fistulation, paralytic ileus and natural diseases such as ulcerative colitis.

Physiological effects of hypovolaemia

Twenty five per cent of the cardiac output flows through the kidneys. Of the total renal flow, 94% passes through the cortex, and the remaining 6% through the medulla. Although the blood supply is the largest of any organ in the body, the kidneys are extremely susceptible to a reduction in their blood supply, a susceptibility made more remarkable by the finding that the oxygen tension in the renal vein is much higher than in all other organs. This would naturally suggest a high oxygen reserve was present, the ratio of oxygen delivery to oxygen extraction being 8% as compared to 65% for the myocardium. The reasons for this are complex but, in practical terms, such is the distribution of blood within the kidney that the medulla – which is subdivided into an outer stripe containing the thick descending loops of Henle and the thick ascending loops of Henle, and an inner stripe which contains the hairpin loop of Henle – exists in a relatively hypoxic milieu. This is proven by the fact that, whilst the entire kidney extracts only 8% of the oxygen available to it, the medulla extracts 80% of available oxygen. The cells most at risk in a hypoxic event are those of the thick ascending loops of Henle. This is because when the blood pressure falls and renal perfusion is reduced, an intrarenal redistribution of blood flow occurs. Blood is shunted from the cortex to the juxtamedullary glomeruli, increasing the blood supply to the medulla and decreasing the delivery of solutes to the thick ascending loops of Henle; their metabolic activity and hence their demand for oxygen are thereby reduced. However, should the hypovolaemia persist, sludging takes place in the medullary capillaries, leading to damage to the cells of the thick ascending loops of Henle which may then be sloughed off into the tubules causing tubular obstruction.

If the hypotensive episode is relatively short-lived or mild, the damage remains confined to the cells of the thick ascending loop of Henle; this leads to an impairment of urinary concentrating power so that when the blood supply is restored, there is a continued filtration of plasma and defective solute reabsorption leading to non-oliguric renal failure.

If, however, the hypotensive episode is more severe and prolonged, the tubular damage becomes more extensive, leading to tubular obstruction and full-blown oliguric renal failure.

Thus, four pathogenic mechanisms are concerned singly or together in the renal dysfunction of acute renal failure:

1. Abnormalities in the glomerular capillary bed leading to a decrease in permeability.
2. Vascular abnormalities leading to a reduction in glomerular plasma flow.
3. Renal tubular obstruction due to cellular oedema or sloughing of the cells.
4. A backleak of the glomerular filtrate across the damaged tubular membrane.

Commonly, there is an interval of some hours between changes in the peripheral circulation and changes in the kidney. As a general rule, the kidney cannot withstand hypovolaemia of such severity that the fall in the systolic blood pressure progresses to a level below that of the normal diastolic pressure of the affected individual for longer than 24 hours. Beyond this time-limit, organic changes develop in the kidney converting the situation from one of prerenal to one of intrarenal failure. However, no specific time-limit can be stated, because much depends on the condition of the kidney prior to the 'insult' and on the presence or absence of contributory causes.

The additional factors which may lead to the development of

intrarenal failure, as opposed to simple prerenal failure, are the presence or release of nephrotoxic substances. These include the following:

1. Haemoglobinuria

The common causes of haemoglobinuria are:

a. Mismatched blood transfusion.
b. Plasma hypotonicity after transurethral prostatectomy.
c. Thermal burns leading to massive destruction of red cells in the area of burning.

Normally, free haemoglobin in the circulation is bound to a specific binding protein, haptoglobin, and only when the level in the plasma exceeds 100–120 mg % does free haemoglobin appear in the urine. However, large amounts of haemoglobin can be intraveneously infused into the circulation of an experimental animal without causing adverse effects on the kidney. When a mismatched transfusion is given, however, it produces a reaction between the patient's antibody and the blood group antigen in the membrane of the donor red cell. The complex thus produced causes intense renal vasoconstriction and hence renal ischaemia. Free haemoglobin is then precipitated in the renal tubules, because the subsequent renal vasoconstriction causes a reduction of the glomerular filtration rate which naturally depresses urine flow.

The treatment of this condition is the immediate cessation of the blood transfusion, if one is being administered, and an infusion of mannitol.

2. Myoglobinuria

The common causes of myoglobinuria include:

a. Crush injuries of the extremities.
b. Sudden arterial occlusion.
c. Severe *Clostridium welchii* infections.

Of these conditions, the effects of a crush injury are the most interesting. The patient may be trapped under debris but, despite suffering severe pain, the general condition may remain good until the crushing agent is removed when, soon after, the affected limb becomes swollen and tense and the blood pressure falls. The haematocrit rises sharply due to massive extravasation of plasma-like fluid into the damaged limb, and oliguria develops due to acute tubular necrosis.

In normal circumstances myoglobin, which is non-toxic, is filtered by the glomeruli and rapidly excreted in the urine. However, myoglobin dissociation products, which are formed in an acid urine, may be directly toxic to the tubular epithelium. Furthermore, myoglobin itself may be precipitated in the tubules causing a physical obstruction to the secretion of urine. This condition is treated by:

a. The immediate administration of sodium bicarbonate in an attempt to increase the pH of the urine and so diminish the formation of the degradation product, ferrihemate.
b. Restoration of the circulating blood volume.
c. The administration of mannitol to improve tubular filtration.

3. Aminoglycosides

The aminogylcosides include streptomycin, kanomycin, neomycin, tobramycin, gentamicin and amikan. Of this group, gentamicin is the most commonly used and remains the treatment of choice for most aerobic Gram-negative infections, although tobramycin is more effective against *Pseudomonas aeruginosa*. All these drugs are potentially nephrotoxic and ototoxic. Gentamicin may cause renal damage if the plasma concentration rises above 10–12 µg/ml, or if the trough concentration (the concentration immediately prior to the next dose) is greater than 2 µg/ml.

Many patients who develop signs of nephrotoxicity have other predisposing factors at work, including advancing age, pre-existing renal insufficiency and infection; this last is, of course, the prime reason for giving the drug.

The cause of the toxic effect is the uptake of the drug by the cells of the proximal convoluted tubules in which the drug accumulates in the lysosomes and inhibits phospholipase activity. Toxicity or necrosis requires seven days of drug administration, but full recovery may follow the cessation of treatment.

4. Radiocontrast media

The mechanism of renal toxicity following procedures such as angiography or computerized axial tomography is unclear, although changes in the renal bloodflow have been shown to occur as also has the aggregation of red blood cells in the glomeruli.

5. Jaundice

It has long been recognized that renal failure is relatively common following operations on patients suffering from obstructive jaundice. In some series, renal failure was responsible for 5% of immediate postoperative deaths.

It had been thought that the important contributory cause was a low blood volume but this thesis has now been abandoned. Investigation has shown that the risk of renal failure is related to the preoperative level of circulating bilirubin, and subsequent investigations suggest that the renal parenchyma is sensitized to changes in blood volume by the presence of high levels of bilirubin glucuronide. The current hypothesis is that bilirubin glucuronide filters through the glomerulus, enters the tubule to form a cast, and exerts a toxic action on the tubular cells.

6. Infection

Infection with Gram-positive or Gram-negative organisms may be associated with the original surgical condition or may follow operation. Organisms of both groups may be nephrotoxic and both may influence the subsequent condition of the patient by converting a normocatabolic into a hypercatabolic state.

7. Hypoxia

The common causes of hypoxia include:

a. Road traffic accidents associated with severe chest injuries.
b. Abdominal or thoracic operations associated with severe chest complications.

Once there has been a gross disturbance of pulmonary function, renal oxygenation, particularly of the medulla, may be reduced below tolerable limits.

Pathological changes in the kidneys

When the oliguria is based purely on a physiological disturbance, no anatomical changes are present in the kidneys. However in more serious cases, two types of lesion can occur: acute tubular necrosis and renal cortical necrosis.

Acute tubular necrosis

In this condition the kidneys are enlarged, and when the kidney is sectioned the surface bulges beyond the capsule due in part to dilatation of the tubules and in part to interstitial oedema. The cortex is pallid in contrast to the medulla, which appears dark and congested.

Histologically, the chief changes are found in the tubules, the glomeruli appearing relatively normal.

In the oliguric phase, the tubular changes are variable and frequently patchy, changes being found more frequently in the distal, rather than proximal, convoluted tubules. As early as three days after the onset of the condition, the cells lining the tubules may become flattened and their cytoplasm basophilic. In areas in which the tubules have been disrupted, the basement membrane may also become fragmented. Brown casts of haemoglobin are commonly seen and, in patients who have suffered a crush injury, myoglobin casts may be prominent. The interstitial tissue of the kidney is grossly oedematous and a large number of cells, including lymphocytes, mononuclear macrophages, plasma cells, polymorphonuclear leucocytes and eosinophils, may be seen clustered around the necrotic and disrupted tubules. As the condition resolves so the cellular debris and the inflammatory cells are rapidly dispersed.

Renal cortical necrosis

Fortunately, this is an uncommon lesion for, unlike tubular necrosis, the condition is irreversible.

Prior to the use of renal biopsy, the condition could only be distinguished from tubular necrosis by awaiting the outcome of the case; if by the fourth week a diuresis had not occurred, it could be assumed that an irreversible lesion was present.

Moderate enlargement of the kidney occurs, and on cut section the cortex is pale yellow except for a thin rim of congested tissue immediately beneath the capsule and another at the corticomedullary junction. Microscopically, the whole of the cortex appears necrotic and the tubules are lined with epithelial cells in various stages of disintegration.

Measures to prevent renal failure

Particular attention should be paid to the following aspects of treatment:

1. Maintenance of a normal blood pressure and blood volume.
2. Prevention of hypoxia.
3. Control of infection.

With regard to the restoration or maintenance of the blood volume, many in the past advocated that at least part of the deficit replacement should be made using Dextran 40 so that intravascular 'sludging' commonly seen in shock would be diminished. The general opinion today favours the administration of blood, human serum albumin or fresh frozen plasma. In a purely prerenal oliguria, the restoration of the blood volume should be followed by a return to normal function of the kidney within 24–72 hours.

Differentiation of physiological from organic oliguria

Several tests will usually distinguish physiological or prerenal from organic or intrarenal oliguria. These include the following:

1. Urine sodium level. When this remains low it indicates that tubular reabsorption and, therefore, tubular function is intact.

2. Blood urea nitrogen to serum creatinine ratio (BUN/Cr). This is normally between 10 and 15:1. A reduction in glomerular filtration from any cause will increase both the blood urea nitrogen and creatinine. However, in prerenal disease due to enhanced reabsorption of sodium and water, the passive reabsorption of urea increases, which in turn increases the ratio to greater than 20:1. A high ratio suggests prerenal disease unless urea production has been increased secondary to some other factor, such as hypercatabolism or parenteral nutrition.

3. Specific gravity. Despite the extreme oliguria which may occur in a physiological disturbance, if the specific gravity remains not less than 1014, it indicates functional activity.

4. Response to volume replacement. When a physiological renal disturbance only has occurred, the adequate replacement of the blood volume should result in an increase in the urine output.

5. Response to mannitol. This is an osmotic diuretic which increases the plasma volume, and decreases blood viscosity and renal resistance. Given in a dose of 100 ml of a 20% solution intravenously after volume replacement in the presence of a prerenal oliguria, the urine output will increase.

6. Response to frusemide. This diuretic acts directly on the renal tubules. It is normally given in a dose of 40 mg. When a negative response occurs to three 'challenges', it must be assumed that organic renal changes are present.

Biochemistry of renal failure

A patient suffering from renal failure is usually described as normocatabolic or hypercatabolic. In the former, the blood urea rises by 30 mg/dl daily (4.7 mmol/l) or less, and in the latter, 60 mg/dl daily (9.4 mmol/l) or more. In addition to the rising blood urea, the plasma concentration of potassium rises. The rate at which hyperkalaemia develops is related to the presence or absence of damaged tissues and the rate of catabolism; the level of 6 mmol/l is regarded as critical since cardiac arrhythmia may then develop followed by peaking of the T waves and later death from cardiac arrest.

Failure to secrete H^+ ions leads to a metabolic acidosis; this may initially be controlled by hyperventilation but will later become uncompensated.

Clinical response to acute renal failure

The total clinical picture in acute renal failure is due to the biochemical disturbances:

1. Dyspnoea. This may be due to fluid overload causing pulmonary oedema, metabolic acidosis or pulmonary infection, occurring either singly or in combination. In the past, fluid overload was the commonest cause of death in this condition.
2. Cardiac arrhythmias which may be due to hyperkalaemia.
3. Nausea, anorexia and vomiting which may be due to water overload or the result of 'uraemia'.
4. Gastric erosions leading to severe gastrointestinal bleeding.
5. Drowsiness and, finally, coma.
6. Infection due to damage to phagocytic activity and immunological systems.
7. Haemorrhagic pericarditis leading to cardiac tamponade.

Principles of treatment of established renal failure

Three relatively recent advances in the field of nephrology have altered the approach to the treatment of acute renal failure. This makes the distinction between the normocatabolic and hyper-catabolic groups somewhat academic, since there is now a greater tendency to progress to haemodialysis early rather than to maintain a strictly conservative regime in the former group of patients. Nevertheless, in areas in which modern haemodialysis units are not yet available or the use of the drug epoprostenol sodium (prostacyclin) is too expensive or is unavailable, it is as well to remember that many patients suffering from normocatabolic acute renal failure can be treated with success by conservative means.

The three advances are:

1. Rapid vascular access via the femoral artery and vein.
2. The availability of modern haemodialysis units.
3. The use of epoprostenol sodium.

As a result of these advances fewer patients are treated conservatively.

The normocatabolic patient

This group of patients can be treated by diet alone. The fluid intake is limited to 400 ml/day, with an additional allocation for insensible water loss which can vary significantly in a patient suffering from a pyrexia or in a hot climate. To reduce the break-down of endogenous protein, 1500 non-protein kilocalories are given daily, usually in the form of Hycal which contains 244 kcal/100 ml. In addition, the daily rise in the blood urea in a normocatabolic patient can be further controlled by the use of anabolic steroids, such as norethandrolone decanoate 50 mg daily by intramuscular injection, which will reduce the rate of break-down of protein by some 40%.

The hypercatabolic patient

Patients in this group, in which sepsis is usually present, are not so easily treated, and dialysis is needed to control the situation. Sepsis must be controlled by antibiotics or surgery or both. Once the blood urea has risen above a concentration of 32 mmol/l, nausea and vomiting may occur which can usually be controlled by chlor-promazine; above this level uraemic fits may occur. If the poten-tially toxic level of potassium is reached, immediate emergency treatment must be instituted, giving an immediate infusion of 100 ml of 50% dextrose together with 10 units of insulin. Once the immediate threat is over, ion exchange resins, such as sodium polystyrene sulphonate, can be used.

Dialysis

The indications vary in different centres but, in general, dialysis is mandatory when the following parameters are exceeded:

1. The blood urea has exceeded 35 mmol/l.
2. The serum creatinine has exceeded 500 mmol/l.
3. The serum potassium has exceeded 6.5 mmol/l, and is not reduced by the measures already described.
4. A significant metabolic acidosis is present associated with the HCO_3 of below is 15 mmol/l.

Dialysis may be performed by either haemo- or peritoneal dialysis, although the former is normally preferred in the surgical patient. In haemodialysis, the patient's blood and the dialysing fluid are brought together, separated by a cellophane or cuprophane membrane only; in peritoneal dialysis, the peritoneum itself is used as a semipermeable dialysing membrane.

The result of either method depends upon the concentration gradient of solutes existing between the blood and the dialysing fluid. Haemodialysis is four times as effective as peritoneal dialysis and, once performed, further dialysis may not be necessary for a further 72 hours. During this time, other aspects of patient care, such as the resetting or nailing of fractures or intensive chest physiotherapy, can proceed.

The disadvantages of peritoneal dialysis in the surgical patient are:

1. It is a fairly lengthy procedure.
2. It is associated with a considerable protein loss.
3. It can only be used when the abdominal cavity is normal.

A fluid exchange of 1–2 l/h is required using an approximately isotonic solution with 1.36% glucose.

Natural history of tubular necrosis

Tubular necrosis begins with an initiation phase in which renal damage is occurring; this is soon followed by the oliguric phase, which may last from a few days to three weeks. At the end of this phase, a diuresis begins – the diuretic phase – during which large volumes of dilute urine are passed. This stage is the equivalent of non-oliguric renal failure. The renal conservation of sodium and potassium is poor during this period, so that the levels of both ions should be carefully monitored; and even though large quantities of urine are being passed, the blood urea may continue to rise before declining. Often, many months pass before renal function becomes completely normal, but it is rare for this condition to end in chronic renal failure requiring long-term dialysis or renal transplantation. However, if the oliguric phase persists for more than three weeks a renal biopsy is required, for this suggests that the condition is one not of tubular but of irreversible glomerular necrosis.

DISSEMINATED INTRAVASCULAR COAGULATION

Disseminated intravascular coagulation (DIC) is also known as: defibrination, consumptive coagulopathy, intravascular coagulation with fibrinolysis and abnormal proteolytic activity.

This condition is defined as one in which there is widespread activation of the coagulation cascade within the circulation resulting in the breakdown of all haemostatic mechanisms – i.e. the coagulation sequence, the platelets, the vessel walls, fibrinolytic mechanisms, inhibitors, kinins and complement systems. In severe cases, fibrin deposition in the microcirculation leads to multiple organ failure.

DIC is never a primary event but is the result of a number of conditions which trigger the process. These may be divided into three major groups:

1. *Tissue activation.* Tissue thromboplastin entering the circulation forms complexes with factor VII, thus activating the extrinsic coagulation cascade. This is the mechanism associated with accidental or major surgical trauma, chemotherapy, malignancy, obstetrical problems, such as premature separation of the placenta, and some snake venoms.
2. *Damage to the vascular endothelium and exposure of collagen.* This situation arises in shock, anoxia, severe

bacterial infections, viraemia and situations in which antigen-
antibody complexes are present in the circulation. In
these conditions, the intrinsic pathway is activated via
factor XII, the Hageman factor, as may be the fibrinolytic
pathway.

3. *Reduced hepatic clearance of activated factors* by the liver. In a
normal individual, the reticuloendothelial system is responsible
for the rapid uptake and clearance of any 'activated' products.
In severe liver disease this mechanism fails and, in addition,
the synthesis of liver-dependent factors falls. Circulating anti-
proteases such as antithrombin II and antiplasmins can be
overwhelmed.

The effect of DIC are catastrophic only when certain modifying
factors are present, the most important of which is blockade of the
reticuloendothelial system, which is normally responsible for
removing many of the triggering mechanisms such as the
endotoxin of Gram-negative bacteria.

Clinical presentation

The disordered haemostatic mechanism in DIC causes the
following:

A bleeding tendency

There is a bleeding tendency frequently from more than one site.
The bleeding may arise from a wound, an area of intestinal ulceration or the uterus. The severity of the bleeding tendency varies
according to the underlying condition. Thus septicaemia, severe
endotoxaemic shock, extensive injury and severe burns nearly
always present with more severe forms of the condition, and when
severe bleeding is present the mortality may reach 100%. The
major cause of bleeding is excessive fibrinolysis, the removal of
formed fibrin clots which is a normal continous physiological
process mediated by plasmin.

The excessive fibrinolysis is related to:

a. Plasmin-destroying factors V and VIII.
b. Plasmin – fibrin – fibrinolysis – fibrin degradation products –
inhibition of platelet function and blood coagulation.

To the surgeon, the underlying cause is usually excessive circulating activator, as occurs in some forms of malignant disease, tissue anoxia and following trauma.

Should the patient survive the immediate crisis multiple organ failure may follow caused either by bleeding or intravascular clotting or a combination of both.

Fibrin deposition may occur in a number of sites:-

(a) In the dermis, causing petechiae, purpura, gangrene and acrocyanosis. In a classic lesion the tissues around an affected vessel exhibit necrosis and haemorrhage without any accompanying inflammation.

(b) In the kidney, in which the rich microvasculature acting as an efficient sieve promotes renal damage.

(c) In the lung, in which the lesions produced lead to the adult respiratory distress syndrome, ARDS, otherwise known as 'shock lung'. The basis of the pathological changes in the lung which lead to such a severe disturbance of pulmonary physiology are, first the deposition of platelet rich microthrombi leading, after the destruction of the platelets, to the formation of fibrin rich thrombi and second the deposition of hyaline membranes both intravascularly and extravascularly in the alveoli and ductuli alveolaris. In addition bleeding into the lung tissue may occur leading to increasing respiratory failure and haemoptysis.

(d) In the central nervous system, causing focal ishaemia or if bleeding occurs more widespread destruction.

In addition red cell fragmentation occurs within the loose fibrin network which is deposited causing anaemia, the so-called microangiopathic anaemia.

Diagnosis

The diagnosis of DIC is made by a combination of features:

1. The correct clinical situation is present.
2. Laboratory investigation reveals that activated products
   are present in the plasma, resulting in disordered coagulation.
3. Secondary fibrinolysis.

Laboratory diagnosis

No single test has yet been described to establish the diagnosis of DIC; this is because of the complex interrelationships between the various components of the coagulation process.

Only the indirect effects of thrombin can be observed, such as:

1. Decreased levels of factors VIII, V and I, due to their utilization and destruction.
2. Intermediate products from the prothrombin molecule will yield a prothrombin peptide which can react with factors X and V and phospolipid in the prothrombin complex, yielding more thrombin and amplifying the system further.
3. The sequence, thrombin – fibrinogen – fibrin causes hypofibrinogenaemia due to fibrin formation. The fibrin may then lyse (secondary fibrinolysis) producing monomers which may inhibit fibrin polymerization and form soluble complexes with fibrinogen or fibrin degradation products.
4. Thrombin may potentiate platelet aggregation resulting in thrombocytopenia and acquired storage pool defects.
5. Factor XIII may be altered or depleted.
6. The plasminogen – plasmin pathway may be activated, resulting in a reduced level of plasminogen, a fall in factor VIII and the release of fibrin degradation products.

Thus the common screening tests for the presence of DIC are as follows:

1. *Prothrombin time* (PT). Normally 13–16 sec, this is prolonged due to reduced levels of factors, V, II, VII, X and I.
2. *Thrombin clotting time* (TCT). The thrombin clotting time is a rapid screening test for the conversion of fibrinogen to fibrin. Thrombin is added to plasma, and the time taken for fibrin formation is the thrombin clotting time. In standard tests using normal plasma as a control, the TCT is 13–15 sec, and is prolonged in DIC due to the reduced concentration of plasma fibrinogen.
3. *Activated partial prothrombin time* (APPT). This test is a development of the partial thromboplastin time, in which the variable of contact activation is eliminated by the addition of an activator to obtain full contact activation. The normal value is 30–42 secs, a time which is exceeded when there is a decrease in factors VIII, X, II, V and I.
4. *Fibrinogen level.* The normal fibrinogen concentration is 2–4 g/l. This level is reduced by virtue of its breakdown by plasmin, with the result that the level of fibrinogen degradation products (FDP), normally in concentrations of less than 5 μg/ml, rises.

5. *Thrombin time.* Normally 13–17 sec, this is prolonged by the decrease in fibrinogen, assuming that no heparin has been given to the patient.
6. *Platelet count.* The platelet count is a very sensitive indicator of DIC, a thrombocytopenia occurring in the majority of cases.
7. *Blood film.* The blood film may show the changes characteristic of microangiopathic haemolytic anaemia, in which fragmented red cells, often triangular or 'pincered' in shape, indicate the tearing or shearing mechanism responsible. Microspherocytes and an obvious thrombocytopenia are common.

Treatment

The first step in the treatment of DIC is to treat, if possible, the triggering mechanism; e.g., in septicaemia by the administration of appropriate antibiotics, in severe blood loss by correcting hypovolaemia, or in acidosis by bringing the pH to more normal levels. However, in only a few cases can the condition be brought under rapid control. In general, time passes before control is achieved. Therefore, effort is directed towards:

1. Restoration of haemostasis.
2. Prevention of microemboli.
3. Removal of existing thrombi.
4. Necessary support of those systems most severely affected.

The restoration of haemostasis is achieved by the transfusion of blood or fresh frozen plasma. The latter is the ideal replacement as it contains all the vitamin K factors as well as factor V, VIII, fibrinogen and ATIII, this last being an intrinsic inhibitor of plasmin activation. Platelet concentrates can also be administered, always remembering that the half-life is 70 hours.

Paradoxically, for many patients the administration of heparin is the treatment of choice. The rationale for this is the inhibition of systemic intravascular coagulation. This treatment produces the most favourable response in haemorrhagic states associated with septicaemia. An initial dose of 50–100 units/kg followed by 10–15 units/kg per hour thereafter is the recommended dose schedule.

Steroids have been used but found to be ineffective, and it has been suggested that if fibrinolytic activity is demonstrated which is difficult to quantify, a drug such as aminocaproic acid may be helpful because this drug is a potent inhibitor of plasminogen. Others believe, however, that aminocaproic acid should never be used because it may foster further intravascular thrombosis. Theoretically, the removal of thrombi once formed could be achieved by the administration of streptokinase, but the danger of bleeding appears to outweigh its advantages.

POSTOPERATIVE PARALYTIC ILEUS

Paralytic ileus may be defined as inadequate peristaltic activity of the gastrointestinal tract; it may be segmental or affect the entire length of the tract. All abdominal operations are normally followed by a period of reduced or absent peristalsis, but usually within 48 hours bowel sounds can be heard with a stethoscope. Shortly afterwards the patient passes flatus per rectum and initially the intestinal activity may be so exaggerated that severe abdominal cramps are felt by the patient.

Illeus as a pathological entity can, therefore, only be recognized if the normal pattern of recovery following an operation is delayed. Such a delay can be anticipated if, at the time of the initial operation, the patient is suffering from a general peritonitis or this complication occurs postoperatively. An additional aetiological factor is undue handling of the gut.

Many investigators believe that ileus results from a reflex, mediated through the sympathetic nervous system, which inhibits the interdigestive motor complexes which normally propel the intestinal contents distally. Such a belief is supported by numerous experiments. Thus, Cannon and Murphy in 1907 showed that ileus could be induced in cats by testicular crushing only if the splanchnic nerves were intact. If the splanchnic nerves were divided prior to the injury, ileus did not occur although paralysis could still be induced by undue local trauma to the gut. Such findings led Cannon and others to the conclusion that ileus was of reflex origin. Further support for the role of the sympathetic nervous system was supplied by Burnstein, in 1939, who found that spinal anaesthesia in humans led to an increase in small bowel activity. Once the lack of forward propulsion has been established, the distension and atony may be enhanced by interference with the blood supply and, possibly, by an intracellular potassium loss.

Treatment

As with many other conditions, prevention is better than attempting to treat the established condition. The improvements in anaesthesia, including the use of relaxant drugs, has led to much less handling of the bowel at operation. The swifter control of infection by the use of antibiotics has also undoubtedly led to a decrease in the number of patients seen with severe ileus.

Conservative treatment has traditionally depended on the administration of moderate but regular doses of morphine sulphate 10–15 mg 6-hourly, and attention to the fluid and electrolyte balance, particularly of the serum potassium. Morphia probably exerts no specific benefit, although it does, experimentally, increase small bowel tone. However, one secondary action of this alkaloid is to reduce the secretion of bile and pancreatic juice, thereby reducing the fluid load which must be moved onwards. Its most beneficial effect is probably its sedative effect.

More specifically, the muscle of the bowel may be stimulated by parasympathomimetic agents. These are divisible into two distinct groups. (1) The true parasympathomimetic agents, such as the cholinesterases, which possess the muscarinic rather than the nicotinic effects of acetylcholine; in this group are the drugs, bethanechol, carbachol and methacholine chloride. (2) The anticholinesterases, which inhibit the enzymatic hydrolysis of acetylcholine by cholinesterase; this group includes the drugs, galantamine hydrobromide, neostigmine and physostigmine, the actions of this last being similar to those of neostigmine but with a more pronounced muscarinic activity. All these drugs have been used with variable results. Of the cholinergic drugs, bethanechol (which is not inactivated by cholinesterase) has been used, but caution must be exercised if the patient is an asthmatic.

In 1971, Neely and Catchpole suggested that the action of the parasympathomimetic agents could be enhanced by blockading the sympathetic inhibition of the gastrointestinal tract. The drugs chosen for this purpose were either guanethidine sulphate, an adrenergic blocking agent interfering with post-ganglionic nervous transmission, or phentolamine mesylate, which is in theory an α-receptor blocking agent. The dose of the former drug is 20 mg given by slow intravenous infusion over 40 minutes, and of the latter, 20 mg given over 20 minutes. Neely and Catchpole reported on a series of patients in whom treatment with these drugs followed by the sequential injection of either bethanechol or prostigmine improved gastrointestinal activity. There is little doubt that parasympathomimetic agents will stimulate both contraction and, sometimes, coordinated peristalsis, leading to the onward passage of bowel contents. However, in some cases, although contractions are powerful enough to induce severe colic, the condition is not relieved. In these rare cases surgical interference may be beneficial.

Two surgical techniques have been advocated. The first, proposed by Wangensteen in 1953, is a simple loop ileostomy, performed through the first available bowel which prolapses through a right iliac incision. The second is to perform an ileotransversecolostomy, an operation first suggested by Handley in 1925. The author has very occasionally used both techniques but prefers the former, as an uncontrollable faecal fistula may follow an ileotransversecolostomy which involves an anastomosis performed under very difficult conditions in a patient who may be in both electrolyte and metabolic chaos.

15 Tracheostomy

INDICATIONS

There are many indications for tracheostomy and they may be classified in a variety of ways. The operation is performed as either a planned procedure, e.g. the formal tracheostomy which accompanies total laryngectomy, or an emergency procedure, e.g. emergency tracheostomy in severe maxillofacial injury. Of all the emergency tracheostomies performed in the past, those performed for the treatment of laryngeal diptheria produced the most dramatic effect diminishing the overall mortality of this disease considerably. The indications for tracheostomy can be grouped under three headings but these differing indications are not mutually exclusive:

1. Indications based on respiratory insufficiency.
2. Indications in which tracheostomy is necessary before or in the course of treatment.
3. Indications based on pharyngolaryngeal dysfunction in which the patient is unable to keep a clear airway.

In clinical practice, the indications for immediate tracheostomy are nearly always multiple; for example, a tracheostomy may be indicated in a patient suffering from multiple injuries for the following reasons:

1. The presence of severe maxillofacial injuries may produce airway difficulties.
2. Injuries to the chest, if severe, result in the increasing retention of bronchial secretions followed by failure of respiratory function. It is, however, present practice to maintain such a patient by tracheal intubation for at the very least several days before peforming a tracheostomy.
3. Respiratory failure following a severe head injury may hasten the onset of, or worsen, cerebral oedema.

Indications based on respiratory insufficiency

This group of indications consists of a large number of different conditions. In many patients, respiratory insufficiency is based on supratracheal airway obstruction, the causes of which may be divided into:

1. Infective.
    a. acute epiglottitis.
    b. acute laryngotracheitis.
    c. acute oedema of the cords caused by the inhalation of 'flash burns.'
2. Mechanical.
    a. carcinoma of the larynx.
    b. post-thyroidectomy haemorrhage if attempts to pass an endotracheal tube fail.
3. Nervous.
    bilateral abductor paralysis of the vocal cords.

In other patients respiratory insufficiency may be caused by central factors:

1. Head injury accompanied by brainstem paralysis.
2. Severe poisoning.
3. Ascending polyneuritis, poliomyelitis, tetanus.

Any patient suffering from respiratory insufficiency should have repeated estimations of their blood gases. Whatever the original starting point for the $Pa\text{CO}_2$, this becomes critical at 80 mmHg (11.0 kPa) and at this level, temporary means of improving respiratory function must be instituted.

MEASURES TO DEAL WITH TEMPORARY RESPIRATORY DIFFICULTY

When the cause of respiratory difficulty is considered to be temporary, the situation may be treated by endotracheal intubation alone. A modern portex tube can be left in situ for about nine days. The larynx and the cords must be carefully inspected at intervals to ensure that oedema and ulceration are not occurring. The advantage of an endotracheal tube over tracheostomy is that the surgical complications of the latter and the resultant scar are avoided.

Disadvantages of an indwelling tube are as follows:

1. It is less well tolerated than a tracheostomy.

2. It is difficult to fix.
3. It may kink in the pharynx.
4. It may be displaced, usually into the right main bronchus.
5. It increases airway resistance.
6. Portex tubes tend to block more readily with inspissated secretions and therefore demand excellent humidification for their management.
7. Pulmonary infection readily occurs if the tube is improperly managed.

If the glottic anatomy is so distorted that an endotracheal tube is very difficult or impossible to pass, an immediate tracheostomy should be performed, since repeated trauma associated with failure to pass a tube will precipitate or aggravate already present laryngeal oedema. Endotracheal intubation itself is not without its complications, but these are seen more commonly in childhood. They include:

1. Glottic webs.
2. Granulomatous reaction.
3. Subglottic stenosis.
4. Inexplicable permanent cord paralysis.

In an emergency in the presence of acute supratracheal airway dysfunction, the cricothyroid membrane can be punctured either by a cricothyrotome or by a large bore needle. This immediately relieves the severe respiratory difficulty so that the subsequent manoeuvre can be performed in less difficult circumstances.

TRACHEOSTOMY TECHNIQUE

The head should be held steady in the extended position by an assistant. This forces the trachea into the most accessible and superficial position. A vertical or limited collar incision in the skin and superficial fat is made after infiltrating the area with local anaesthetic. The collar incision is made some 2 cm below the cricoid cartilage. The author advises a vertical incision for the inexperienced operator since it makes subsequent steps in the operation much easier.

The deep cervical fascia and the plane between the two muscle bellies of sternohyoid is divided, and a small self-retaining retractor inserted to spread the margins of the wound. A search is now made for the isthmus of the thyroid which is identified and divided, if necessary, laying bare the first, second, third and fourth tracheal rings. The first and the second are left undisturbed; the third and fourth are divided. In the past, when a major indication for tracheostomy was the relief of a diptheritic stridor, it was as well at this point to be sure that the eyes were out of the way of the inevitable globule of sputum which would be coughed out through the opening for, if lodged in the eye, this could lead to a diptheritic infection. An early postoperative complication of tracheostomy is early displacement of the tube. If only an ordinary window is cut, without any further action, the tube is difficult to reinsert soon after the operation should it become dislodged. To overcome this difficulty, the trachea can be opened in a T-shaped manner, suturing the angles of the T to the skin. Alternatively, an inverted U-shaped incision can be made in the trachea, the apex of the U then being sutured to the skin.

Once the trachea is opened, either a double lumen silver tracheostomy or a plastic cuff tube is inserted and the attached tapes are fastened behind the neck, taking care that they are neither too loose nor too tight. If they are too loose, the tube will have a tendency to fall out of the wound when the neck is flexed.

The type of tube used depends somewhat on the indications for the tracheotomy. If the primary indication for tracheostomy is, for example, the respiratory difficulty associated with a 'flail chest', a cuffed Portex tube is required because an essential feature of the management of such a patient is continous positive pressure ventilation. If, however, the tracheostomy is to be of very temporary nature and is required to relieve simple airway obstruction, then a silver tracheostomy tube can be used. This consists of three parts: an outer tube, an inner tube, and an obturator which fits into the outer tube and which is used by the operator to slip the tube into the trachea after it has been opened. Once the tube is in position, the obturator is removed and the inner tube is inserted; this can be removed at intervals and cleansed.

A tracheostomy reduces the dead space in an adult by approximately 140 ml and also allows freer access to the bronchial tree for removal of secretions. However, the dead space normally warms and humidifies inhaled air and it is important that both functions are replaced by some artificial device, otherwise the cilia of the tracheobronchial mucosa lose their mucous covering and become inactive. This leads to the accumulation and inspissation of secretions on the inner wall of the endotracheal tube, the distal trachea and the bronchi.

Once the tracheostomy is in place, an air/oxygen mixture is given. The inspired air/oxygen tension should, however, be no greater than that which will maintain the arterial oxygen tension at between 80 and 100 mmHg (10.6–13.3 kPa), because if oxygen is inspired at a Pao_2 greater than 300 mmHg (40 kPa) for longer than 36 hours, retrosternal discomfort and cough may occur (the Lorrain Smith effect).

The continuous administration of pure oxygen may eventually lead to bronchopneumonia and death. The mechanism of oxygen poisoning is unknown, but it is generally believed that such high oxygen levels interfere with surfactant formation in the alveoli.

Complications of tracheostomy

Complications of tracheostomy are not infrequent. A retrospective study performed in Oxford some years ago showed that out of a total of 389 patients some form of complication occurred in 252 and that 13 deaths were directly attributed to the operation. The important complications include:

1. *Pulmonary infection.* This is the most frequent complication of tracheostomy and special care is needed to avoid it. Sterile plastic and endobronchial catheters should be used for bronchial toilet, and these should be passed by personnel trained in aseptic techniques using, if possible, disposable sterile plastic gloves. Frequent bacteriological examination of the sputum is required, and care should be taken to prevent the accumulation of secretions.
2. *Displacement of the tube.* Displacement may be dangerous in the first few days preceding the development of a proper track. Later, angulation of the metal tube may lead to erosion of the trachea and the innominate artery, resulting in severe haemorrhage and death. Alternatively, backward displacement of the tube may lead to oesophageal damage.
3. *Air embolus.* This hazard usually occurs at the time of the operation.
4. *Surgical emphysema.* This ensues when the skin around the tracheostomy tube is so tightly sutured that air cannot escape from the neck.
5. *Subglottic stenosis.* This occurs if the first, or possibly the second, tracheal ring is damaged. If they are divided or eroded, chondritis of the cricoid cartilage may develop which can lead

to total collapse of the airway and the need for a permanent tracheostomy.

6. *Crusting of the tube and bronchi*. Inadequate humidification of the inspired air leads to the accumulation of inspissated secretions which may block the tube.

7. *Granulomata of the trachea*. These form proximal to the tracheostomy opening and cause a ball valve obstruction at the upper lip of the stoma which gives no trouble until the tube is removed.

8. *Late tracheal stenosis*. This is caused by ischaemic necrosis of the tracheal rings by a cuff tube, and can be prevented by releasing the pressure in the cuff for a few minutes every few hours.

9. *Pneumothorax*. This is due to injury of the dome of the pleura when performing the initial operation.

Tracheostomy in the infant

Emergency tracheostomy in the infant is seldom necessary, but if it is required there are certain aspects of the operation which are dissimilar to the operation in an adult. A window should not be cut in the trachea which should merely be opened by a longitudinal incision in the second and third rings. When the tracheostomy is to be maintained for some time, the Liverpool type of silver tube should be used, which has an inspiratory valve at the end of a side opening. The object of such a tube is that whilst the baby inspires through the tube, it expires through the fenestration, the air being forced through the larynx, thus ensuring that this develops properly.

16 Diagnosis and treatment of blunt injuries of the abdomen

INTRODUCTION

Although this discussion is chiefly concerned with the problem of blunt injuries to the abdomen, it is important to recognize that abdominal trauma is associated with injuries outside the abdominal cavity in nearly three-quarters of all patients admitted to hospital. This is because one of the commonest causes of abdominal injury is the road traffic accident, during which the four major systems – craniospinal, chest, abdominal and skeletal – may all sustain severe damage. It is this fact which has led, in the United Kingdom, to the compulsory wearing of seat belts for the driver and his front seat passenger, and this will shortly be extended to include passengers sitting in the rear seats as well. However, legislation has not yet been passed to make the wearing of seat belts compulsory for high speed coaches.

In the highly developed Western countries, nearly one-half of all deaths between the ages of 15 and 29 years are the result of injuries on the road. Surveys performed on trauma victims in the United Kingdom and elsewhere have indicated that some 20% of deaths are preventable, and that if injuries to the central nervous system are excluded this figure rises to nearly 65%. The chief causes of death are failure to stop bleeding, failure to prevent hypoxia and a delay in surgical intervention.

All the major systems are interlinked and each, when injured, may exert an adverse effect on the others. Thus, when the chest is so badly damaged that hypoxia and hypoxaemia follow, there is a detrimental effect on the brain, particularly if this organ has also been injured. Partially damaged brain cells, which might have recovered if fully oxygenated, die, and there is also considerable evidence that hypoxia hastens the onset of cerebral oedema or worsens established oedema. Alternatively, severe haemorrhage leading to hypovolaemic shock, particularly in the presence of hypoxaemia, may finally result in cortical or tubular necrosis of kidneys which were previously normal.

ESSENTIAL STEPS IN MANAGEMENT

1. Airway obstruction. A common cause of death after severe blunt injury to the abdomen is airway obstruction. A patient injured just after a heavy meal may vomit, producing a mechanical block to respiration if aspiration occurs. Such a patient requires an immediate bronchoscopy to have any chance of survival. The vomiting of fluid contents from the stomach which are then aspirated may lead to progressive pulmonary dysfunction due to the adult respiratory distress syndrome (see Ch. 13). The tongue may block the upper airways either by falling backwards in a patient who has been rendered unconscious or by backward displacement in a patient suffering from a concommitant fracture of the lower jaw.

Although the airway may be free, an associated chest injury may lead to gross and increasing pulmonary dysfunction which may necessitate the passage of a cuffed endotracheal tube and positive pressure ventilation.

2. Haemorrhage. A second common cause of death following an abdominal injury is haemorrhage followed by hypovolaemic shock. If severe, as for example from a ruptured aorta, this may cause either immediate or almost immediate death from cardiac failure; if less severe but untreated, it may cause delayed death from failure of other vital systems.

Even closed fractures may lead to the loss of large volumes of blood: a fractured pelvis may cause the loss of 3–4.5 litres, a fractured humerus 1–2.5 litres. The 'expected' blood loss can be approximately judged from clinical examination. If this volume is than replaced but no satisfactory haemodynamic response occurs, it is reasonable to assume, in the absence of previous cardiac disease or severe chest or brain injury, that there is internal bleeding the source of which must be identified and treated as soon as possible.

When difficulties are encountered in resuscitation, a central venous line should be inserted and, if available, a Swan–Ganz flow-directed balloon-tipped pulmonary catheter; this, when 'wedged' into the pulmonary artery, reflects left atrial pressure and the function of the left ventricle. In the 'free' unstabilized position it still permits a reasonable assessment of left ventricular function. Blood used in an emergency should be of the patient's own group or, if unavailable, Group O Rhesus-negative. If plasma substitutes are given, blood for grouping and cross-matching should be taken before they are administered. Initial attempts to resuscitate the patient should be followed by frequent observations of the pulse rate, blood pressure, central venous pressure, left atrial pressure, the state of consciousness and the pupil size and reaction. If the patient is breathing by means of a respirator, a record must be kept of the rate, tidal volume, inspired oxygen concentration and peak pressure. If the patient is ill enough to require intensive care, a narrow catheter will usually be passed and the urine output monitored in this way.

SIGNS ASSOCIATED WITH ABDOMINAL INJURY

Certain external signs may be present when the abdomen has been injured. Thus, the presence of tyre marks or extensive bruising on one or other side of the chest or upper abdomen may suggest that the liver or spleen or both, have been injured. Similar marks across the centre of the abdomen are frequently associated with injuries to the bowel, mesentery and, particularly, to the mesenteric vessels.

Plain X-rays of the abdomen may show fractures of the lower rib cage: if present on the left side, the spleen may well be injured; fractures on the right are consistent with an injury to the liver. Free air may be found, indicative of injury to a hollow viscus.

One clinical problem to which there is no solution is to distinguish between the pain and tenderness of an injury which involves only the abdominal parietes, and one which involves an internal viscus. In most cases, the diagnosis of intraperitoneal haemorrhage becomes obvious so long as the patient suspected of having sustained such an injury is carefully monitored, since finally he or she develops a rising pulse rate and a falling blood pressure.

INVESTIGATION

1. X-rays

Plain abdominal and chest X-rays should be taken. Fractured ribs on the right indicate the possibility of a ruptured liver, and fractures on the left a possible injury to the spleen. Air in the abdomen indicates rupture of a hollow viscus and loss of the psoas shadow a retroperitoneal haemorrhage.

2. Peritoneal tap and lavage

The use of peritoneal tap for the diagnosis of intra-abdominal haemorrhage was first described by Saloman in 1906. It is only of use when there is sufficient free fluid in the abdomen to permit a specimen to be aspirated. Although this technique was gradually extended from a single site tap made in the region of the umbilicus to a 'four quadrant' tap, this method is no longer used for the diagnosis of intra-abdominal haemorrhage. It has now been abandoned in favour of peritoneal lavage, since it was found that simple aspiration was positive in fewer than 20% of patients in whom less than 200 ml of blood was present in the abdominal cavity, and that even in the presence of 500 ml positive results could be achieved in only 80% of patients.

Peritoneal lavage, a much more accurate technique, carries a much higher rate of positivity, yields fewer false-negative results and, if carefully performed, virtually no false-positive results.

Method

The method as described by Gill in 1975 is as follows:

1. The bladder is emptied if necessary by preliminary catheterization, after which a nasogastric tube is passed and the stomach also emptied of its contents.
2. The skin and abdominal parietes in the region of the umbilicus in the midline are infiltrated by local anaesthetic. A small incision about 2–3 cm long is now made in the sub-umbilical region and the peritoneum exposed. The peritoneum is picked up with forceps and a purse string suture inserted, after which a small incision is made through which a dialysing catheter or a multiperforated polythene tube is inserted into the abdominal cavity.
3. The purse string suture is now closed around the catheter and isotonic saline – in children 500 ml and in adults 1000 ml – is slowly introduced into the peritoneal cavity with the patient in a slight Trendelenberg position.
4. After 10 minutes, the fluid is syphoned from the cavity and any

bloodstaining is regarded as indicative of intraperitoneal haemorrhage.

Not all serious blunt injuries of the abdomen can, however, be diagnosed by this method, since it requires that bleeding must have occurred within the abdomen itself. Thus, retroperitoneal haemorrhage from the pancreas or kidneys may cause profound hypovolaemia but is not necessarily associated with a positive lavage.

3. Computerized axial tomography

With the increasing availability of computerized axial tomography, this method has become of particular value in the investigation of those patients suffering from blunt trauma to the abdomen in whom injury to the liver, spleen, pancreas and kidneys is suspected. It is now being used in some centres not only to confirm the diagnosis but also to determine treatment.

4. Ultrasonography

Whilst computerized axial tomography may not be generally available, the majority of hospitals are now equipped with ultrasonography, an investigation sufficiently sensitive to pick up subcapsular splenic haematomata and renal injuries.

HEPATIC INJURIES

Hepatic injuries are sustained in approximately 15–20% of blunt injuries to the abdomen; grit, burns or bruises on the right upper abdomen and lower chest may be found, and in older patients fractured ribs on the right. In children, the chest is so elastic that any degree of intra-abdominal catastrophe is possible without the ribs being broken. Abdominal tenderness is present in 70% of patients, and abdominal rigidity is also common. Rebound tenderness and rigidity may spread if intra-abdominal bleeding and bile leakage continues after the initial period immediately following the injury. Severe haemorrhage will, of course, lead to hypovolaemic shock.

The chief causes of death following hepatic injury are bleeding, the direct result of the injury itself or delayed bleeding due to a reduction in the platelet count and deficiences of factors V and

VII; the depletion of the platelet count depends on the volume of blood given, and the deficiency of the factors to the degree of hepatic injury.

Classification of severity

Many different classifications of liver injury have been described and by the use of computerized axial tomography, if available, an extremely accurate picture of the severity of the injury can be obtained prior to surgical treatment; this is an advantage when considering the means by which access to the damaged organ should be achieved.

Four basic degrees of liver injury are recognized:

1. A simple superficial laceration from which bleeding will probably have ceased at the time of laparotomy.
2. Deeper lacerations involving the liver parenchyma only, which are usually bleeding at the time of laparotomy.
3. Severe burst injuries associated with severe parenchymal destruction and injury to major intrahepatic vessels, the treatment of which will require wide debridement.
4. Severe injuries in which extrahepatic vessels such as the hepatic veins are torn or avulsed from the inferior vena cava.

Fortunately, 85% of liver injuries fall into the first category and are not of themselves associated with any mortality. Approximately 10% fall into the second category and may be associated with some mortality, possibly due to infection followed by secondary haemorrhage. Only 5% fall into groups 3 and 4, in which a mortality of at least 50% can be expected.

Very occasionally, the liver remains intact but the common duct is avulsed from the porta hepatis.

Treatment

Minor injuries

When laparotomy reveals one or more superficial lacerations of the liver, bleeding will nearly always have ceased by the time the patient is submitted to surgery. Assuming that there is no other injury, a drain can be put down to the area of liver damage and removed a few days later when it is obvious that, barring the onset of infection and a secondary haemorrhage, no further problem exists. If bleeding is continuing when the abdomen is explored, the liver wound should be sutured by using interlocking horizontal mattress sutures, inserting each suture approximately 2 cm from the edge of the wound. Special absorbable tampons are now generallly available through which the stitches can be inserted and which diminish the danger of individual stitches 'cutting out'.

Severe lacerations

Severe lacerations of the liver will be associated with severe bleeding. This can be controlled temporarily by compressing the damaged lobe between both hands. Unfortunately, although this manoeuvre will stop the bleeding if it is from the liver alone and thus allow the patient to be resuscitated, as soon as the pressure is released bleeding commences once again.

Before proceeding further, an attempt must be made to distinguish this type of injury from those in which damage to the hepatic veins has occurred. This can sometimes be achieved by compressing the vessels in the free edge of the lesser omentum between finger and thumb, a manoeuvre first described by Pringle in 1908. If bleeding continues after compressing or clamping these vessels, it suggests that the retrohepatic vena cava or the hepatic veins themselves have been damaged.

Assuming this manoeuvre appreciably reduces the volume of bleeding, what further operative procedure should be performed? The alternatives are as follows:

1. Obviously avascular liver tissue can be removed and the bare area packed. This method is subject to the following disadvantages:

   a. a pack does not necessarily control the bleeding.
   b. there may be fatal haemorrhage when the pack is removed.
   c. the pack itself may produce pressure necrosis.
   d. secretions and exudate have difficulty in draining and as a result severe intrahepatic and subphrenic infections may develop.
   e. biliary fistulae may develop.

2. The obviously devitalized liver tissue on either side of a major laceration may be removed, after which the 'fissure' is packed by an omental flap which is fashioned from the greater omentum, supplied by the right gastroepiploic artery and drained by the right gastroepiploic vein. This pack is inserted

into the laceration and the edges of the liver are loosely brought together by liver stitches as described. The proponents of this method claim that by using an omental pack the dead space of the wound is eliminated, and that tamponade produced by the pack controls minor venous bleeding. The critics of this method suggest that one may be leaving in situ a devitalized mass of liver parenchyma.

3. On the basis of these criticisms it can be argued that the correct treatment is to remove that part of the liver lying lateral to the major laceration, using the finger fracture technique first described by Lin. This method leaves undivided vessels intact and these can be ligated as they are exposed. Vessels already divided as a result of the initial trauma are transfixed if possible in the substance of the liver. Following removal of the liver tissue it is occasionally possible to secure haemostasis by removing the peritoneum from the under surface of the diaphragm and then suturing it onto the raw surface of the liver. The author has been able to use this technique on only one occasion but it worked!

Complex liver injuries

Complex liver injuries with laceration of the lobar branches of the portal vein, the retrohepatic vena cava or the hepatic veins are relatively rare following blunt trauma to the abdomen, but are relatively common following gunshot wounds.

The performance of an anatomical lobectomy does not appear to lower the mortality. In this regard, it should be noted that the original division of the liver into right and left lobes was by reference to the attachment of the falciform ligament and the fissures for the ligamentum teres and venosum. However, Hjortsjö showed, on the basis of the segmental branching of the bile ducts, hepatic artery and portal vein within the liver, that the functional division of the liver into its two major lobes is considerably to the right of these attachments. On the superior surface of the liver there is no superficial marking to indicate this division, but on the inferior surface this boundary is indicated by a line extending from the gall bladder fossa towards the inferior vena cava. The plane between the two lobes forms an angle of about 35° with the vertical plane, and 20° with the sagittal plane.

The chief difficulty in this type of injury is to control the haemorrhage. In order to gain access to a severe injury, the abdominal incision should be converted into a thoracoabdominal approach by dividing the costal margin; alternatively, the incision may be extended upwards in the midline and a sternotomy performed using a Sarn's saw. Proponents of the latter method make the point that when the pericardium and diaphragm are divided, the inferior vena cava is easily exposed above the entry of the hepatic veins after which the subhepatic cava can be isolated and controlled. However, in the author's very limited experience, total control of the suprahepatic cava so reduces the venous return to the heart that the patient collapses forthwith and the anaesthetist demands the restoration of some bloodflow.

If the classic thoracoabdominal approach is made, division of the right triangular ligament allows the liver to be rotated. If the bleeding is coming from the right hepatic vein it will often be controlled by this manoeuvre alone, after which the tear in the vein can be identified and sutured; the damaged liver tissue must then be removed.

In order to maintain venous return, various authors have described the insertion of temporary caval shunts. However, these appear to be associated with no reduction in mortality, perhaps because when this manoeuvre is deemed necessary other complications defeat the surgeon. Indeed, if hepatic resection is required, mortality rates slightly in excess of 50% have been recorded.

One of the great difficulties facing the surgeon dealing with very severe hepatic injuries is undoubtedly the torrential haemorrhage which accompanies them. Once the volume of blood transfused exceeds 12–14 units, the bleeding time is prolonged and a haemorrhagic state develops. To prevent the inevitable thrombocytopenia, one unit of fresh blood should be given for every 4–5 units of banked blood and if there is already an abnormality platelet concentrates are necessary. Within the liver biloma and abscesses may develop, but these can now be treated by interventional radiography in most cases, a tube drain being inserted under direct vision using ultrasonic means of identifying the lesion.

SPLENIC INJURIES

Rupture of the spleen following blunt injuries to the abdomen is more common if the spleen is already abnormal; a malarial spleen is especially prone to rupture following relatively mild trauma, as also is the spleen of a patient suffering from leukaemia or infectious mononucleosis.

The majority of splenic injuries consist of lacerations which run across the convex outer surface, but occasionally the spleen is totally shattered or completely avulsed from its pedicle.

Diagnosis

The clinical diagnosis should be suspected when the patient develops signs of internal haemorrhage associated in the elderly with fractures of the left lower ribs. Abdominal rigidity will develop which will extend down the left side of the abdomen either slowly or rapidly according to the severity of the bleeding. Referred pain in the left shoulder will occur, and the patient may be tender on rectal examination. In a minority of patients abdominal signs never develop, although a peristently high pulse rate together with a mild pyrexia and a low haemoglobin should alert the surgeon. It is in this type of case, in which the condition is unrecognized, that a massive delayed haemorrhage may occur. The incidence of this complication is unknown; the various reported series indicate that it may occur in as many as 35% of patients, although in the author's experience other incidence figures quoting 2% seem nearer to the truth.

Various theories have been advanced to explain the condition. One theory is that if the diagnosis is not made the omentum walls off the laceration and so prevents further bleeding, but this does not explain why a patient may develop such a dramatic haemorrhage some days later. A second, more plausible theory, is that there is delayed haemorrhage only when the original injury produces a small laceration of the tail of the pancreas. Under these circumstances, the membrane enclosing the haematoma is presumed to be gradually digested away by the pancreatic enzymes until finally it gives way, permitting a further bleed to occur.

The diagnosis of splenic injury may be reached on clinical grounds and confirmed as the source of bleeding either by radionuclide scanning or, more accurately, by computerized tomography following the injection of iodine.

Several investigators using the latter have drawn up grading scores according to the severity of the injury. One such, described by Mirves and Whiteley in 1989, defined the following four grades of splenic injury:

Grade I   —Capsular avulsion, superficial laceration or

subcapsular haematoma less than 1 cm in depth or diameter.

Grade II —Parenchymal lacerations of 1–3 cm in depth. Central or subcapsular haematomata of 1–3 cm in depth.

Grade III —Lacerations greater than 3 cm in depth. Central or subcapsular haematomata greater than 3 cm in diameter.

Grade IV —Fragmentation.

Treatment

The best method by which injuries to the spleen should be treated has been a matter of considerable debate over the past two decades.

Splenectomy

In 1911, Kocher stated that injury to the spleen demanded excision of the organ, that no evil effects would follow and that the dangers associated with bleeding would be effectively curtailed.

Although, in 1919, a paper was published showing that asplenic rats had a diminished lifespan and an increased susceptibility to infection, this knowledge went unnoticed until 1952, when King and Schumaker of the Toronto Children's Hospital reported that five children in whom a splenectomy had been performed for the treatment of congenital spherocytosis had developed severe pneumococcal infections which had resulted in two deaths. Since that date, the incidence of infection following splenectomy has been repeatedly examined. A study of 688 children and adults who had undergone splenectomy for trauma showed that the mortality rate from infection was 0.58%, as compared to the 0.01% expected in the normal population; the mortality rate after splenectomy was thus some 58 times higher than expected. A further paper, in 1984, in which 604 asplenic adult patients were studied showed that 10 patients had suffered severe infections, although none had died.

This increased susceptibility to infection is due to the part played by the spleen in the defence against bacterial infections. The spleen is a major producer of IgM antibodies, and in children under one year of age IgM levels fall after splenectomy and remain low for about one year before returning to normal. More importantly, there is an immediate and prolonged fall in the plasma tuftsin level, an important factor concerned with the ability of the polymorphonuclear leucocytes to phagocytose encapsulated bacteria such as the pneumococcus.

In addition to its immunological role, the spleen is also concerned with red cell maturation – moulding the reticulocytes and reducing the membrane surface by about one-third, converting them into biconcave discs typical of the mature red cell.

A very late complication of splenectomy is a two-fold risk of developing ischaemic heart disease, possibly due to a decrease in the deformability of the erythrocytes and an increase in blood viscosity.

Thus, despite the danger that failure to perform a laparotomy and remove the spleen might lead to the neglect of other associated intra-abdominal injuries and the possibility of delayed haemorrhage, the feeling has developed that, if possible, splenic tissue should be preserved and so in recent years a much more conservative approach to splenic injuries has become popular.

Alternatives to total splenectomy

In a recent Norwegian trial of 147 patients admitted with a splenic injury, 43% did not undergo operation and in 64% of the whole series the spleen was saved.

In many centres, especially those equipped with CAT, the scan is used to make the diagnosis. However, the decision to perform a laparotomy is based on purely clinical gounds – the extension of physical signs or a decreasing haematocrit being taken to indicate the need for surgery. In one American series, 87% of patients selected for non-intervention were successfully treated without operation.

If, however, a laparotomy is indicated, a number of techniques other than a straightforward splenectomy are available.

1. When dealing with less severe injuries in which a subcapsular haematoma is present, the capsule should be stripped from the surface of the spleen, the haematoma drained and haemostasis obtained by the use of microfibrillar collagen AVITENE or Gelfoam which may be incorporated into the sutures. An alternative to this method is the intraparenchymal injection of fibrin glue; local application is not very satisfactory if the wound is bleeding fiercely because the glue tends to be washed off before polymerization takes place.

2. *Splenorrhaphy*. In some more serious injuries the removal of devitalized material is required. This can be accomplished by the performance of a partial splenectomy or a hemisplenectomy due to the segmental nature of the blood supply to the spleen: in the majority of individuals there are two primary lobar intrasplenic branches, so that an upper or lower pole splenectomy can be accomplished by the finger technique after ligation of the appropriate major vessel.

3. *Splenectomy and autotransplantation*. If exploration reveals that splenectomy is inevitable, autotransplantation has been suggested as a means of preserving some splenic tissue and thus avoiding the dangers of infection. In the majority of reported series, some 50 g of splenic tissue is harvested and divided into 5-mm thick slices. The greater omentum is then opened and the slices placed between the two layers. The function of the transplanted tissue can be demonstrated by:
   a. Splenic scans.
   b. Following the morphology of the red cells.
   c. Quantitative estimations of IgM antibody.

However, the degree of protection against the pneumococcus remains dubious, because it has been shown that such protection is only present if the main arterial supply to the organ is intact. There have been several reports of postsplenectomy sepsis in patients suffering from splenosis, this latter being one of the late complications of injury to the spleen due to the scattering of splenic cells within the abdominal cavity. If this occurs, it tends to produce adhesions within the abdomen and recurrent attacks of intestinal obstruction.

SMALL BOWEL INJURY

Blunt injuries of the small bowel are caused by a number of mechanisms, including:

1. The gut is crushed against the vertebral column.
2. Shearing injuries occur causing disruption of the blood supply.
3. Shearing injuries cause disruption of continuity between fixed and mobile points, i.e. at the duodenojejunal flexture and at the ileocaecal junction.

Presentation and treatment

When disruption of a major vessel occurs the patient may present with hypovolaemic shock and the signs of peritoneal irritation. The realization that an intrabdominal catastrophe has occurred is usually obvious, and laparotomy is therefore indicated as soon as resuscitation has been completed. The disrupted blood vessels, which will nearly always have ceased bleeding by this time because of the shearing nature of the injury, must be identified and tied off. Close attention must then be paid to the extent of the ischaemic bowel which must be resected.

When the disruption involves only the bowel wall, the diagnosis may not be immediately obvious. A small laceration of less than 1–2 cm may be sealed off by neighbouring coils of bowel and the omentum, and go undiagnosed until the developing intra-abdominal abscess ruptures into the general peritoneal cavity. However, if an area of abdominal tenderness associated with rigidity and rebound tenderness persists, exploration is indicated in order to close the perforation.

A somewhat more dangerous situation arises when the only injury is an intramural haematoma. It may be many days later before the bowel wall ruptures either as a result of ischaemic changes or of infection or both.

RENAL INJURIES

Renal injuries are usually produced by blows on the flank or across the lumbar region. A severe blow liable to be complicated by renal injury is frequently associated with skeletal injury particularly to fractures of the transverse processes of the lumbar spine.

Presentation

The commonest presenting symptom is haematuria, which is likely to occur in all patients except those in whom the kidney has been completely avulsed from its pedicle. In addition, if a severe cortico-medullary laceration has occurred a gradually increasing swelling in the loin and even in the abdomen may develop and become palpable, followed later by bruising.

Investigation

A variety of investigations are available to establish the diagnosis.

Plain X-rays of the abdomen may reveal a soft tissue mass obliterating the psoas shadow, an elevated diaphragm or the associated skeletal injuries.

Intravenous pyelography may show total or partial functional impairment and the presence of intrarenal or extrarenal extravasation. Most important of all, it will demonstrate the presence of a normally functioning kidney on the unaffected side, a matter of great importance since the author has seen one case of a child in which a solitary but damaged kidney was removed.

Ultrasonography will reveal the presence of renal haematomata, and if a CAT scan is available an extremely accurate picture of the damaged kidney can be obtained.

Treatment

Injuries in which moderate but rapidly diminishing haematuria occurs, and in whom the IVP shows little change from normal or a generalized diminution of function, require no active treatment.

The treatment of injuries in which investigation shows that a corticomedullary laceration has occurred with extensive extravasation remains a matter for debate.

Some surgeons would argue that when intravenous pyelography shows only the presence of intrarenal extravasation, exploration is unnecessary; whereas it extrarenal extravasation is present, exploration is mandatory. At operation, the kidney should be repaired: either pole is removed and the damaged calyces sutured, after which the polar tissue can be trimmed so that the renal tissue can be opposed. Such treatment avoids the possibility of renovascular hypertension in the future. Other surgeons would argue that even if dye is seen to extravasate from the kidney the patient can still be treated conservatively, so long as an increasing swelling does not develop in the loin. It is in this group that a pararenal pseudohydronephrosis may slowly develop due to the extravasated blood and urine slowly occluding the pelviureteric junction.

If the kidney is either shattered or avulsed, nephrectomy is required. In the latter, haematuria may be very transient, since the secretion of urine ceases immediately after the injury. Furthermore, although a mass may form in the loin because of the initial haemorrhage, it may not continue to expand since both the renal artery and vein are liable to constrict. In general terms, in the absence of devastating haemorrhage the majority of renal injuries can be treated conservatively; in one series in which 77 patients suffered non-penetrating injury of the kidneys, only 5 were explored.

PANCREATIC INJURIES

Traumatic lesions of the pancreas caused by blunt trauma to the abdomen rarely occur in isolation.

It is not uncommon for pancreatic injury to be missed because there may be no dramatic features to suggest its presence either before operation or when the abdomen is opened. However, if a haematoma is present in the root of the transverse colon, in the periduodenal area or at the duodenal flexure it should be explored.

When the haematoma is present in the periduodenal area, an extensive Kocher's manoeuvre is required so that both the anterior and posterior aspects of the head of the pancreas can be inspected. If the haematoma is in the base of the mesocolon, access to the pancreas can best be obtained through the gastrocolic omentum and the lesser sac; whilst a haematoma in the region of the tail of the pancreas requires that the spleen be mobilized and brought forward.

Treatment

When the pancreatic injury appears trivial and little or no secretion occurs from the organ after an injection of secretin, or no gross lesion of a major duct can be demonstrated by an 'on table' pancreatogram, all that is required is to drain the area.

If, however, a severe laceration of the left half of the pancreas has occurred, the simplest and safest procedure is to perform a distal pancreatectomy which usually demands a simultaneous splenectomy. The major pancreatic duct is ligated and the edges of the pancreas oversewn. A large drain should be brought out into the flank in such a position that if a pancreatic fistula develops the efflux can be readily controlled by an adhesive appliance, attempting to protect the skin between the wound and the rim of the flange with a competitor such as dried milk or by Stomahesive. One further treatment can be tried aimed at reducing the volume discharged from the fistula, should one develop. Because of its effect on bicarbonate, the drug, acetazolamide will reduce the secretion of high volumes of pancreatic juice but, regrettably, has no effect on the concentration of the more dangerous proteolytic enzymes. However, the mere reduction of the volume output makes the fistula easier to manage.

Another drug with a profound effect on pancreatic secretion is glucagon; this has been shown to reduce not only the volume but also the amount of proteolytic enzymes secreted.

When the laceration involves the head or the right side of the gland, the problem is more difficult and the correct management a matter for debate. Fortunately, such injuries are rare. The following procedures have been sugggested:

1. *Pancreatoduodenectomy.* This is a formidable operation carrying a high mortality in an already severely injured patient. If is, of course, followed by insulin-dependent diabetes and exocrine enzyme deficiency.
2. *Extended distal pancreatectomy.* Such a resection can be carried out up to the left border of the portal vein.
3. If the injury is actually in the head of the pancreas an internal Roux loop can be constructed bringing the free end of the loop up to the head and securing it around the site of the injury. This is made easier when the duodenum is also lacerated since at least one edge of the circumference of the loop can be sutured in the manner of an intestinal anastomosis. The jejunum distal to the duodenojejunal fistula is then anastomosed end-to-side into the Roux loop to complete the operation. The author has no personal experience of this method and cannot therefore comment on its efficacy.

17 Diagnosis and treatment of closed and penetrating injuries of the chest

The overall incidence of nonpenetrating wounds of the chest has diminished in the United Kingdom due to the compulsory wearing of seat belts, although other causes of such injuries, e.g. industrial accidents, remain. The incidence of penetrating wounds, however, has increased as violent crime becomes more common.

PHYSICAL EXAMINATION

The physical examination of an individual suffering from a closed injury of the chest may reveal a variety of physical signs.

Inspection may reveal: the presence of gross subcutaneous emphysema due to air leaking from the damaged lung through the pleura into the tissues of the chest wall and beyond; paradoxical respiration; obvious signs of hypovolaemic shock if massive haemorrhage has occurred within the chest; rapidly increasing dyspnoea if a tension pneumothorax is developing; or filling of the neck veins if cardiac tamponade is developing.

In lesser injuries, palpation may reveal merely local crepitus at the site of a fractured rib or local subcutaneous emphysema. Other physical signs may be found on percussion: hyper-resonance in the presence of a pneumothorax, dullness to percussion due to a haemothorax, or a combination of both if a haemopneumothorax is present. Breath sounds may be absent, crepitations or obvious areas of bronchial breathing may be found.

In any event however slight the injury a plain postero-anterior chest X-ray is required.

Chest X-ray

The chest X-ray, so important in the management of a chest injury, should be taken if possible with the patient in the erect or sitting position, since lying flat the full significance of the injury may not be appreciated. For example, in the presence of a haemopneumothorax, a film taken in the lying position may not reveal the true state of affairs since the radiotranslucency of the air within the pleural cavity may cancel the radiodensity caused by the accumulated blood and, furthermore, the anticipated fluid level will not be apparent.

When there is an indication to place a tube in the chest, repeated X-rays should be taken to make certain that the condition has stabilized and that no other features are appearing on the X-ray which might suggest that the injury is more serious than was first anticipated. Other than blood and air in the chest cavity, the plain X-ray may show loops of bowel if a traumatic rupture of the diaphragm has occurred, widening of the mediastinum indicating a traumatic rupture of the aorta, or air in the posterior mediastinum indicating a traumatic rupture of the oesophagus, a condition which can be verified by a gastrografin swallow.

TREATMENT

Less serious injuries

Less serious injuries, such as a fracture of one or two ribs in which investigation shows that the lung has not been punctured producing a pneumothorax, require no treatment other than the administration of analgesics. The chest may be strapped but the result is more cosmetic than useful; it may, indeed, be harmful in the elderly, when such treatment may lead to collapse and pneumonia, particularly in the presence of concomitant pulmonary disease. Pain can usually be relieved by mild or intermediate analgesics, but if these do not appear effective, regional nerve blocks can be performed: a long-acting local anaesthetic agent, such as Marcaine, is injected just lateral to the paravertebral muscles, first in the segment of the fractured rib and then one or two nerves above and below. Pain-relieving measures other than analgesics consist of continous epidural analgesia, or inhalation analgesia using Entamox. This is a mixture of 50% nitrous oxide and 50% oxygen, delivered by the demand principle, the gas not flowing unless a negative pressure is applied to the inspiratory port.

PNEUMOTHORAX

No immediate treatment is required for a small pneumothorax. Few symptoms will be present, and the important factor is to repeat the X-ray after several hours to make sure that it is not becoming more extensive. If, however, a large pneumothorax is present, the pneumothorax is increasing in size or respiratory distress is developing, an intercostal drain must be inserted. When a tension pneumothorax is present, indicated by rapid deterioration of the patient's condition with the development of tachypnoea and respiratory distress, urgent treatment is required. A wide-bore needle thrust through an intercostal space into the pleural space will be rewarded by a rush of escaping air and an immediate improvement in the patient's condition. Following such emergency treatment, the needle should be removed and replaced by an intercostal drain using the technique described below.

Insertion of an intercostal drain

The safest and easiest site in which to insert an intercostal drain is through the second intercostal space anteriorly in the mid-clavicular line. A chest X-ray should be taken as near to the time of insertion as possible in order to verify the presence of air, otherwise damage to the underlying lung may occur. Using the mid-clavicular line as the site of penetration avoids the possibility of injury to the internal mammary vessels, the superior vena cava and the ascending aorta.

The operation is carried out with the patient sitting more or less upright, well supported by pillows. The skin followed by the underlying tissues are infiltrated with a local anaesthetic, making sure to infiltrate the parietal pleura to avoid the rare but fatal complication of 'pleural shock', which the author has seen on one occasion only lead to sudden death in an otherwise healthy man.

A small incision is now made in the skin, after which a suture is passed across the incision and loosely tied at its ends, its purpose being to close the skin wound when the drain is finally withdrawn. A sterile trocar and cannula of appropriate size are then inserted through the incision and thrust through the chest wall into the pleural cavity. The trocar is removed and a plastic drain with a radio-opaque marker and multiple side holes is threaded through the cannula into the chest. The cannula is then withdrawn and the tube connected to an underwater seal. A second suture is then inserted through the skin and wound several times around the catheter, before trying it to prevent it slipping out of position. A dressing is applied around the site of the incision and the patient allowed to adopt whichever position he feels is most comfortable. Once the drain is correctly placed, a stream of bubbles should issue from the underwater tube as the lung expands. Once the bubbling has stopped, if all is well, the fluid level will continue to oscillate with respiration. A plain X-ray should now be taken to confirm that the desired result has been achieved. The tube should then be clamped and left in situ for a further 24 hours before removing it, taking one further X-ray prior to its removal .

Complications

1. The tube may accidently be pulled out of the chest, usually due to the patient being lifted in bed without prior removal of the safety pin normally used to anchor the tube to the bedclothes.

2. The fluid contents of the underwater seal may inadvertently be siphoned into the chest. This can only occur if the bottle is raised to a higher level than the patient. To prevent this, the tube should be clamped prior to moving the patient e.g. if the patient has to be taken to the X-ray department or operating theatre.

3. The tube may become blocked. The simplest explanation of this is that the tube has become kinked between the patient and his bedclothes, but it may also become blocked by clot or exudate.

4. Air may continue to escape from a small laceration for several days but if the lung remains expanded, eventual sealing of the leak will occur. If excessive amounts of air are leaking from the lung, it may be necessary to apply suction to control the situation and obtain satisfactory expansion of the lung. This should be applied at a relatively low pressure 5 mmHg, to the air outlet of the water seal drainage bottle. Only rarely do the above measures fail to procure expansion of the lung and eventual cure of the condition, but if the patient is clearly losing more air from the drain with each breath than his normal tidal volume, a large air leak or a ruptured bronchus is probably present and thoracotomy is indicated.

Chronic pneumothorax

Very occasionally, a patient may present some weeks after a chest injury, suffering from a undiagnosed pneumothorax which has failed to be reabsorbed because of the layer of fibrin which forms over the surface of the visceral and parietal pleura. In this case, whilst drainage should be attempted it will usually be unsuccessful and, in order to achieve re-expansion, a thoracotomy followed by decortication of the lung is required. In removing the 'peel', consisting of coagulum and young granulation tissue, from the surface of the visceral pleura, small leaks will inevitably be produced which must be dealt with by leaving an underwater drain in situ at the end of the operation.

TRAUMATIC HAEMOTHORAX

Bleeding into the pleural cavity may come from a variety of sources. If severe, it may lead to hypovolaemic shock as well as respiratory difficulties, since in the average adult each hemithorax can accomodate up to 3 litres of fluid. A small haemothorax may cause no symptoms, no physical signs and escape notice even on a plain X-ray of the chest, since 200–500 ml of fluid may be hidden behind the dome of the diaphragm and thus escape detection by an X-ray taken in the erect position. If for any reason the chest X-ray is taken with the patient supine, the blood accumulates in the paravertebral area and produces a 'ground glass' appearance over the affected lung field.

Treatment

In the majority of cases, early intercostal drainage, using a drain of reasonable size, 26 Fr gauge, is the most appropriate treatment in order to pre-empt clot formation blocking the tube. The drain should be inserted through the sixth interspace in the mid-axillary line, placing a smaller drain in the second intercostal space in the mid-clavicular line if a pneumothorax is also present.

In the majority of patients, once the blood has been evacuated (this may amount to 1–2 litres) the bleeding stops, since the pulmonary circulation is a low-pressure system, and no further action is required. Beal and his coworkers found that of 694 patients suffering from a traumatic haemothorax, 552 were adequately treated by tube drainage alone, 49 required a thoracotomy and in 42 of these patients there was an associated cardiac lesion. However, should large volumes of blood continue to escape from the chest, to reaccumulate or hypovolaemic shock develop, an indication for thoracotomy exists.

In some patients, a missed haemothorax or the incomplete evacuation of a recognized haemothorax leads to incomplete inflation of the lung due to the formation of a gelatinous matrix on the pleural surface. If this occurs, a thoracotomy is indicated in order to decorticate the affected area of pleura.

FLAIL CHEST

When two or more ribs are fractured in two places or are fractured posteriorly with sternochondral dislocation anteriorly, a 'flail chest' is produced. In this condition, the unstable fragment is sucked in during inspiration and out during expiration with the result that the patient may be unable to create a negative intrapleural pressure and, consequently, the tidal volume falls, the degree being determined by the size and instability of the flail segment. In consequence tachypnoea develops and, in serious injuries, anoxia and hypercapnia ensue to be followed by exhaustion and death.

A 'flail chest' rarely occurs in isolation. In order to produce such an injury – which in the past in the United Kingdom was most commonly due to impaction of the chest against the steering wheel in road traffic accidents – great forces are required which may result in the development of a pneumothorax, haemothorax, lung contusion or even rupture of great vessels.

The immediate 'first aid' treatment of such an injury consists of rolling the patient onto the side of the injury. This has the effect of controlling to a limited extent the degree of paradoxical movements of the flail segment, allowing the patient to take deeper and more effective breaths.

Following admission to hospital and an assessment of the situation as regards concomitant injuries, attention must be turned to respiratory function. The need for treatment directed at improving ventilatory capacity is indicated by a rising $Pa\text{CO}_2$ – a level above 35 mmHg (4.6 kPa) is considered unacceptable in the very young, whereas a level below 55 mmHg (7.3 kPa) may be quite acceptable in the elderly – and a falling $Pa\text{O}_2$. In severely ill patients, the $Pa\text{O}_2$ may fall to 40 mmHg (5.0 kPa) compared to the normal of 100–110 mmHg (13 kPa).

Two methods of improving ventilatory capacity are currently in use:

1. *Prolonged positive pressure ventilation*. This method was first

introduced in 1956 by Avery, who used the term 'internal pneumatic fixation' to describe it. Using this method may require several days in an intensive care unit before the chest is sufficiently stable to permit spontaneous respiration and, whilst the method yields extremely satisfactory results in younger patients, it is associated with a high mortality in the elderly.

2. *Internal fixation* using Kirschner wires or Rush nails to fix the broken ribs. Whilst this method appears to have some advantages in the elderly, its use is restricted by the presence of concomitant diseases or injuries which make a prolonged operation undesirable. Furthermore, even in the best hands, fixation of the affected ribs is often difficult, if not impossible, due to the degree of comminution.

Whichever method of treatment is adopted, intensive physiotherapy is required including endobronchial catheter suction in order to diminish the retention of secretions and so reduce the incidence of infection.

PULMONARY CONTUSION

In addition to obvious injuries to the chest wall, some degree of pulmonary contusion occurs. This lesion was first recognized in 1909 by Payne, who drew attention to the fact that such a lesion could develop without any apparent external injury. The lesion may vary from a single small area of damage, accompanied by localized oedema and extravasation of blood, to multiple or conglomerate areas of widespread damage. In the latter situation, the radiological picture is one of large areas of frank consolidation. The condition may only become obvious some 24 hours after injury, the first clinical evidence being the development of tachypnoea and the finding of wet râles on physical examination. A constant accompaniment of lung contusion is haemoptysis and excessive tracheo-bronchial secretion. From the point of view of lung function, compliance diminishes and arteriovenous shunting occurs. Treatment must be directed towards improving oxygenation and preventing the onset of infection.

Intermittent positive pressure ventilation via an endotracheal tube ensures that the work of respiration is reduced and that secretions can be aspirated. Such treatment is not directed at the lesion itself but to the remaining functioning lung.

TRAUMATIC RUPTURE OF THE DIAPHRAGM

This injury may be missed, since the force required to rupture the diaphragm is such that the injury is seldom isolated and attention is therefore directed to the associated injuries. Because there is no hernial sac, the abdominal viscera pass freely into the chest. Of particular interest is herniation of the stomach, since a dilated stomach lying within the chest cavity may be mistaken for a loculated pneumothorax and a chest drain inadvertently put into it. Injury to the right hemidiaphragm may cause little in the way of symptoms or signs because the liver rarely herniates upwards.

The diagnosis is usually made on the plain chest X-ray and, if doubt exists, contrast studied will confirm or refute the diagnosis.

The laceration should be repaired and the abdominal contents returned to the abdomen using either a left seventh intercostal space thoracotomy or an upper left paramedian incision. Care is taken to examine all the viscera in this area, particularly the spleen which may be ruptured as well. The crura are not involved. The tear normally radiates from the junction of the tendinous and the muscular portions of the diaphragm and is usually very easily repaired.

CLOSED INJURIES OF THE HEART AND GREAT VESSELS

Nearly all such injuries are almost immediately fatal, the patient dying of cardiac tamponade, heart failure or hypovolaemic shock.

Should a cardiac injury be suspected, the patient's condition should be carefully monitored. The clinical picture indicating that cardiac tamponade is occurring consists of increasing venous pressure, rapidly developing hypotension, tachycardia and muffled heart sounds. If the blood pressure is taken throughout the whole of a respiratory cycle, it will be found that the decline in the systolic blood pressure during inspiration is much greater than normal, a physical sign known as 'pulsus paradoxus'.

The X-ray shows the cardiac shadow to be enlarged with a rather globular appearance, although in some patients the X-ray will show minimal changes even though the patient's condition is deteriorating. In such patients, echocardiography will demonstrate the presence of fluid in the pericardium.

The immediate need in this situation is to relieve the intrapericardial pressure. This can be achieved in the first place by pericardiocentesis, which can be performed in a number of ways:

1. By inserting a wide-bore needle alongside the xiphisternum
    and angulating it upwards into the pericardium.
2. By inserting a needle through the fourth interspace, close to
    the sternum in order to avoid damage to the internal
    mammary artery and vein.
3. By making a small midline epigastric incision and dividing the
    central tendon of the diaphragm.

When blood is found, the chest should be opened by an incision
made from the left sternal edge to the anterior axillary line
following the curve of the fifth rib. The fourth interspace is then
entered and the internal mammary artery and vein are tied off
before extending the incision over its full extent. Thereafter, a
tense blue pericardium is seen which confirms the diagnosis. The
pericardium is opened and the myocardium exposed, after which
any visible laceration is sutured.

Rupture of the aorta may also follows a closed chest injury, the
laceration normally occurring at the level of the ligamentum
arteriosus or at the diaphragmatic hiatus. In patients reaching
hospital, the rupture commonly involves the intima and the media,
continuity of the vessel being retained by the intact adventitia
which, for a time at least, may withstand the intra-aortic pressure
before giving way to form a false aneurysm.

A radiograph in a classic case will show widening of the
mediastinum, but careful examination is needed to observe this
since many other radiographic signs may be visible due to the
various lesions present in the chest.

If the condition is suspected, the diagnosis can be confirmed by
aortography or ultrasonography after which a thoracotomy should
be performed and, using one of a variety of bypass techniques or
moderate hypothermia, the affected segment of the vessel replaced
by a graft. Eighty five per cent of such patients suffering from
major trauma to the heart or great vessels die; the remaining 15%
may be saved if operated upon in time.

PENETRATING WOUNDS OF THE CHEST

Penetrating wounds of the chest present an even more dangerous
situation than do uncomplicated closed injuries since, in addition
to the chest wall and lungs, other intrathoracic structures such as
the heart and great vessels are more commonly injured by this
means, and associated damage to the abdominal organs may occur

if the causal agent penetrates the diaphragm. An apparently uncomplicated stab wound delivered below the nipple line in any axis might for example, if the individual is in full expiration at the moment of injury, result in injury to the liver, spleen, stomach or even the colon, for the simple reason that the domes of the diaphragm may ascend to a higher level than the nipples during this phase of respiration.

Even small wounds of the chest may produce a life-threatening situation in the form of a sucking pneumothorax. In this condition, a valve-like entry into the pleural cavity permits air to be sucked into the pleura during inspiration but fails, due to the valve-like effect of the wound, to allow air to escape from the wound during expiration. The result is a tension pneumothorax and a life-threatening situation.

The immediate treatment is to place an occlusive dressing over the wound to prevent more air being sucked into the wound, after which an intercostal drain should be inserted through the second interspace using the technique already described. Once the respiratory condition is controlled, a decision can be made regarding debridement of the wound, when dead tissue, loose fragments of bone will be removed and the skin wound closed, if necessary by using rotation flaps.

Following relief of the critical condition and the treatment of hypovolaemic shock, preparations can be made for an exploratory thoracotomy.

18 Burns and scalds

INTRODUCTION

Between 400 and 500 people in England and Wales die annually from the effects of major burns, mostly children and old people. Factors which increase the incidence of burns and scalds include:

1. *Age*
   a. In the majority of children under three years of age the injury is a scald, caused either by a hot water bottle bursting in the cot or the accidental tipping over of a pan or kettle containing boiling water.
   b. After the child has learnt to walk a large percentage of burns are caused by 'backing up' against an open coal or gas fire when wearing inflammable night attire.
   c. During the adult's working life the majority of major burns and scalds are caused by industrial accidents.
   d. In adults over 60 years of age, momentary cerebral ischaemia based upon cerebral atherosclerosis or arterial spasm becomes common.
2. *Disease*
   a. Epilepsy.
   b. Cerebral atherosclerosis.
   c. Alcoholism
3. *Occupation* Individuals dealing with industrial processes requiring heat are liable to burns and scalds, e.g. foundry workers or laundry workers. Regardless of their cause the two most important problems in the management of burns and scalds are, (a) resuscitation and (b) the treatment of the resulting wound.

Factors affecting the outcome of a burn or scald include:

1. Age—extensive burns or scalds at the extremes of age are

much more serious than those occurring in healthy adolescents or young adults.
2. Depth of the injury.
3. Inhalation of noxious fumes. Whether this has occurred at the time of burning can often be deduced from the appearance of the patient and the history of the incident leading to the injury. Burns taking place in a closed environment are frequently associated with inhalation injury. The nasal vibrissae may be singed and there may be an obvious laryngitis.
4. Pre-existing cardiopulmonary disease.

RESUSCITATION

The major factor indicating the need for resuscitation is the area of the burn or scald, as this determines the volume of fluid and protein loss.

Area of burn or scald

The area can be assessed from the 'Rule of Nine', first devised by Polaski and Tennison but often referred to as Wallace's rule. This divides the body surface into areas, the head and neck being equal to 9% of the total body surface, the anterior surface of the trunk 18%, the posterior surface 18%, each lower extremity 18%, each upper limb 9% and the perineum 1%. Note that the surface of an individual's hand with the fingers extended is equal to 1% of the body surface of an adult. Although the rule is accurate enough for clinical purposes it is not in fact a true measurement of the various parts of the body since the percentages of each area change relative to one another as growth occurs. Thus, the relative surface area of the thigh and leg increases with growth whereas that of the head and neck decreases. To correct for the difference in area in children, the child's age in years is subtracted from 12 and the resulting number added to the figure for the adult head and neck or subtracted from the figure for the lower limbs.

In a child, the critical area of a burn or scald is usually considered to be 9% and in the adult, 15% excluding the erythema; if the area involved is greater than this, intravenous therapy should be commenced as soon as possible. This is to prevent the development of hypovolaemic shock since immediately after the burn or scald is sustained there is a loss of both fluid and a plasma-like material from the burnt surface. Some of this fluid may appear on the surface and be temporarily contained in blisters whilst much leaks from the damaged capillaries into the interstitial tissues in which it is sequestered. This loss is greatest in the first 24 hours and ceases within 48 hours. In an adult, approximately 1 litre of plasma is lost for every 10% of the body surface burnt or scalded.

Erythema is not initially taken into account in estimating the area burnt, but may have to be included later as blistering develops.

In addition to fluid and plasma loss, when the burn exceeds 10% of the total body area the loss of red cells becomes important.

Depth of burn or scald

The depth of a burn or scald is also important from two points of view.

1. Depth determines the magnitude of the red cell loss. This is because:

a. The deeper the burn the greater the degree of haemolysis of the red cells following direct exposure to heat.

b. The greater the depth of the burn the greater the entrapment of red cells by thrombosis in blood vessels within the area of the burn.

c. The morphology of the erythrocytes passing through the damaged area is so altered that they are subsequently sequestered and prematurely destroyed.

d. Red cells are lost by sludging.

2. Depth determines the time taken for healing to occur.

Many elaborate tests have been described to measure the depth of a burn or scald but none have proved satisfactory. The majority depend on the injection of dyes into the circulation when the damaged area having lost its blood supply fails to be stained. Unfortunately in the hours following a severe burn or scald a progressive deterioration of the small blood vessels in the immediate area occurs expanding the area of tissue damage despite the apparently normal circulation in the immediate post-burn phase.

The clinical history may be extremely helpful, however, in that electric burns are usually full thickness and uniform throughout whereas scalds, unless caused by immersion tend to be more superficial; and flash burns vary in depth across the injured area. However the passage of time alone reveals the depth of a burn or scald, since a partial-thickness injury will heal within 2–3 weeks whereas a full-thickness injury remains covered by a raised eschar beneath which is active granulation tissue.

Water loss

Loss of skin leads to increased water loss from the body surface by evaporation. Normally, in a temperate climate this loss is approximately equal to 15 ml/m^2 per hour whereas in the presence of a full thickness burn it may rise to some 200 ml/m^2 per hour. This evaporative water loss is accompanied by a corresponding heat loss, each gram of water evaporated from the body surface representing a loss of approximately 0.575 kcal. Since evaporated water is virtually sodium free, an underestimation of the rate of loss may rapidly result in the development of hypertonic dehydration due to hypernatraemia.

Other indications for intravenous therapy

Other indications that intravenous therapy is required include:

1. A deterioration in the general condition of the patient.
2. A rising pulse rate.
3. A falling blood pressure.
4. A fall in the urine output.
5. A fall in cardiac output. In all severely burnt patients an immediate fall in the cardiac output occurs which is thought to be due to an as yet unidentified myocardial depressant. Assuming the patient survives, after adequate resuscitation, the cardiac output returns to normal within 36 hours.
6. A rising haematocrit which indicates the degree of haemoconcentration consequent on the plasma loss. In the past the measurement of the haematocrit was the keystone to many methods of calculating the volume of plasma necessary to restore a normal circulating blood volume.

Fluid Replacement

Three types of fluid can be used to replace the exudate.

Saline or Ringer lactate

Interest in the use of saline in the treatment of burns requiring resuscitation was largely stimulated by the high cost of plasma. Some 30 years ago it was shown that normal saline could be used almost as satisfactorily as plasma in adults but was associated with a higher mortality in children. The theory on which the use of crystalloid is based is that filling the extracellular space with isotonic saline increases the tissue pressure and so prevents leakage from damaged capillaries and also that sodium loss is the chief cause of burn shock. Practically, an advantage of Ringer lactate over normal saline is that the acidosis associated with the infusion of excessive chloride ions does not occur.

In the United Kingdom the Birmingham Burns Unit tested this method of resuscitation in both children and adults and concluded that it was satisfactory only when the patient was closely supervised so that a change to plasma or HPPF could, if necessary, be made.

Nevertheless, some centres believe that colloid replacement is of little benefit during the first 24 hours following a burn, due to the generalized capillary changes which extend throughout the whole circulatory system rather than being confined to the area of the burn itself. Thus, in these centres it is considered that saline alone should be given in the first 24 hours followed by colloid replacement thereafter when the generalized effect of the burn has resolved.

2. Human purified protein fraction (HPPF)

HPPF contains 90% albumin, has the same sodium content as plasma and a potassium content of 2.3 mmol/l. It does not require reconstitution but is expensive.

3. Dextran 110

If Dextran is used, blood should be taken for cross-matching prior to its administration. Rarely the infusion of Dextran is associated with anaphylactoid reactions at the commencement of the transfusion or allergic phenomena such as headache, fever or a rash somewhat later.

In the United Kingdom plasma protein fraction is now the most commonly used replacement fluid although each burn unit has its own variation. Many formulae have been devised to calculate the volume required; that proposed by Muir and Barclay is adequate.

Firstly the area burnt or scalded is assessed by the Wallace rule of nine. The greatest period of exudation occurs during the first 12 hours after which the rate declines over the next 24 hours. This total period is divided into six periods of 4, 4, 4, 6, 6 and 12 hours. The volume required is the same for each period and can be calculated from the following simple formula:

$$\frac{\text{Percentage area of burn} \times \text{weight in kg.}}{2}$$

The first aliquot of HPPF must be given within the first 4 hours and even if the transfusion does not begin until, say, 3 hours after the injury, the calculated total volume required should be given in the remaining hour.

In addition to HPPF, 100 ml of water hourly should be given by mouth if the patient does not find it nauseating, or intravenously if oral feeding is impossible.

If Ringer lactate is used, greater quantities of fluid are required using the Baxter and Shires formula of 4 ml/kg per 1% area burnt and administering one half the total volume in the first 8 hours.

Furthermore, if the burn is larger than 20% of the total body surface blood is necessary in addition to plasma, the volume required being equal to 1% of the patient's blood volume for each 1% of the burn area. The approximate blood volume can be calculated from the following simple formula:

$$\text{Blood volume} = \text{weight in kg} \times 75$$

After the theoretical requirements have been calculated a number of other factors should be considered. Note should be taken that young children and elderly adults will not tolerate excessive quantities of fluid, that patients suffering from pre-existing cardiovascular or renal disease should be treated with caution, and that in flash burns, in which respiratory tract irritation may be present, pulmonary oedema is commonplace. Furthermore, extensive burns are often followed by paralytic ileus, and in these patients fluids should not be given by mouth until bowel sounds return.

Assessment of resuscitation

Clinical evidence suggesting that resuscitation is progressing satisfactorily is provided by the following data:

1. The patient is calm.
2. Peripheral circulation returns.

3. The blood pressure returns to normal levels.
4. The pulse rate remains steady.
5. Urine output is satisfactory.

In a child, the urine output should be 7 ml/hr or more, and in an adult 25 ml/h or more. The urine should be routinely tested for haem pigments; organic renal failure seldom occurs if there are no haem pigments in the urine, but if they occur renal failure remains a possibility in the early stages.

If the urine output falls, the specific gravity of the urine should be measured since this provides a rough guide to the renal concentrating power. Other tests follow those described in the section on renal failure.

Following resuscitation, it should be remembered that a negative nitrogen balance follows a severe burn or scald. To overcome this, an intake of at least 20 g of nitrogen is required for every square metre of the surface area of the burn during the first month, and 15 g thereafter until complete healing has occurred. If rapid closure of the wound is obtained by appropriate grafting techniques this loss can be greatly reduced. In addition to nitrogen, adequate calories are required giving 25 kcal/kg bodyweight plus an additional 40 kcal for every 1% of the surface area of the burn. To give such a large number of calories may require enteral feeding by means of an indwelling nasogastric tube of fine bore giving a solution containing 1.5 K cal/ml with an osmolar concentration of not more than 600 mosmol/l. In addition adequate vitamins should be given.

CLASSIFICATION OF BURNS OR SCALDS BY DEPTH

Unfortunately, there is at present no agreed standard international classification of the depth of burning or scalding. The National Research Council of Canada simplified what had been a somewhat complex situation by recognizing only two degrees of burning:

1. *Partial-thickness loss*, which implies that the deeper epithelial elements are alive and that epithelialization will take place without the need for grafts.
2. *Full-thickness loss*, which implies that there has been complete destruction of all epithelial elements. Such a burn cannot heal from surface elements but only by the ingrowth of epithelium from the peripheral margin, aided, possibly, by contraction.

Interestingly this classification corresponds to that used by Giovanni di Vigo some 500 years ago.

One clinical test of burn depth is pin-prick sensation. This was first described by Dupuytren in 1832 but has recently been judged to be somewhy unreliable. The appreciation of pinprick as pain does not disappear until there is necrosis in a plane just superficial to the deepest sweat ducts. Deep partial thickness burns (Jackson's Classification) are associated with a reduction in sensation or analgesia; deep dermal burns and full thickness burns are totally analgesic. To perform the pinprick test properly the skin should be pricked firmly in several places to the square inch to be sure that analgesia is present. If appreciation to pin prick is sharp, healing will occur within three weeks with no loss of skin texture.

A much more sophisticated classification based on the skin elements from which a burn may heal has been proposed by Jackson and others of the Birmingham Accident Hospital's Burn Unit. The classification requires an elementary knowledge of the structure of normal skin and takes account of the following five principles:

1. It is based upon the depth of necrosis, not on the intensity of the surface burning.
2. It should relate the depth of burning to the critical plane of the deepest epithelial elements.
3. The type of burn should be capable of early diagnosis.
4. The classification should have a prognostic significance indicating:
    a. whether skin grafting will be necessary.
    b. the probable type of scarring.
5. The classification should include all the depths of burning commonly distinguished and referred to in clinical practice.

To apply a classification that obeys these five principles requires an elementary knowledge of the normal structure of skin. With the exception of some special sites, which include the scalp, beard, palms and soles, the undersurface of the dermis is composed of a deeper layer of collagenous fibres that cross each other to form an extensive feltwork of rhomboid meshes in which the main direction of the fibres runs parallel with the skin. Through the mesh formed by the fibrous septa, fat from the subcutaneous tissues proper bulges up into the deeper layers of the corium to form domes of varying height. The two specialized elements of the skin, the hair follicles and sweat glands, take origin at different depths; the former arise in the lower dermis and at the very most merely penetrate the summit of the fat domes, whereas the sweat glands penetrate more deeply so that many of them take origin deep in the fat domes even below the level of the rhomboid network of collagen fibres. Some distance deep to the sweat glands is the horizontal, subdermal arterial and venous plexus.

So far as a burn or scald is concerned, any burn that still leaves the remnants of most of the hair follicles and sweat ducts can heal, if properly treated, in about 14 days, whereas if all the hair follicles are destroyed, but a full complement of sweat glands remains, healing will require 21 days. Burns deeper than this, but still possessing some sweat gland remnants, can heal of themselves but the process will be slower. This type of burn has been termed the deep dermal burn, and anything deeper than this in which all epithelial elements have been destroyed is full thickness.

Jackson's classification of burns based on the depth of necrosis is given in Table 18.1

Table 18.1   Classification of burns based on depth of necrosis

1	Erythema	No loss of epidermis	Hyperalgesia
2	Partial thickness skin loss:		
	Superficial	No loss of dermis	Hyperalgesia
	Intermediate	Healing from hair follicles	Normal or hypoalgesic
	Deep	Healing from sweat glands	Hypo- or analgesic
3	Deep dermal burns	Scanty epithelial foci which may or may not epithelialize the surface under the conditions prevailing	Analgesia
4	Whole skin loss	Healing from edge only	Analgesia

Partial skin loss, although easily divisible into three subgroups on anatomical grounds, cannot easily be distinguished immediately after burning, and this is so also for the deep dermal burn, the various levels of burning becoming apparent only with the passage of time.

A full thickness burn may, however, be readily diagnosed: the presence of exposed fat, muscle or bone in the depth of the burn leaves no doubt of its severity, as also does the more common brown, somewhat translucent appearance of the skin traversed by thrombosed veins. Simple erythema, with or without blister formation, usually indicates a partial thickness burn, but it should be remembered that the more extensive the burn the more likely it is that some parts will be full thickness.

TREATMENT OF THE BURN ITSELF

Small full thickness burns

Burns produced by direct contact with a hot object, molten metal or an electric heating element can be excised and grafted as soon as they are first seen.

The extensive burn

There are four possible methods of managing the larger burn.

1. *By occlusive dressings and late grafting*

This method may be used for any burn. If occlusive dressings are applied it is essential that the chemical used on the dressing should neither macerate the tissues nor damage viable epithelium. Many different antibiotics, either alone or in combination, have been used. More recently silver nitrate and silver sulphadiazine have been introduced. The advantage of the latter is that it prevents early invasion of the burn by *Pseudomonas aeruginosa*. After the maximum exudative period is over, the dressings can be left undisturbed for periods of between three and five days. Whatever the antibacterial compound used, a burn dressing should isolate the burn from the environment and be absorptive and bulky enough to ensure that exudate does not reach the outer layers of the dressing. Superficial burns heal within 10–20 days. Ungrafted deep dermal burns, in the absence of infection, may heal within 25–30 days. Full thickness burns require to be excised and grafted after making sure that bacterial contamination is minimal in degree and that a *Haemolytic streptococcus* is not present.

2. *Open Method*

This method of treatment is ideal for superficial burns, for burns of the face or burns involving only one aspect of the circumference of a limb. Normally prior to exposure the burn is cleansed. The exudate of a partial thickness burn dries with 48–72 hours forming a crust under which epithelial regeneration occurs, and in 14–21 days the crust separates spontaneously, leaving an unscarred well healed surface. When all layers have been destroyed the dead skin becomes a thick tough eschar with its surface lying at the level of the intact skin. As this dries it contracts eventually lying below the surface of the surrounding healthy skin. The eschar slowly loosens, but the speed at which it does so is dependent upon bacterial growth and the natural development of granulation tissue at the interface between the eschar and the underlying tissue.

At some point a decision must be made to excise the eschar and after suitable preparation of the granulating surface apply split thickness grafts.

In place of split thickness grafts which inevitably leave an ugly scar, attempts have been made to seed the recipient area with epithelial cells grown in culture from cells obtained from the recipient.

In children suffering from extensive burns the principle of 'tiger' grafting has been employed, alternating strips of skin obtained from the mother with strips obtained from the child itself. An alternative dressing is pigskin.

One advantage of obtaining total skin cover, however temporary, is the reduction of sepsis and a lessening of the catabolic phase which follows severe burning.

3. Immediate extensive excision

Extensive excision followed by immediate grafting of whole thickness massive burns soon after injury has been subjected to extensive trials in many centres in the hope that such radical treatment would reduce the mortality. This has not been achieved and the method has been abandoned.

4. Tangential excision

Tangential excision followed by immediate grafting (Fig. 18.1) was a technique initially described by Janzekovic in 1968 and in 1975 he reported his results in 4370 patients.

It can be used when examination of the burn shows that analgesia to pinprick is present since this indicates, according to the classification introduced by Jackson, that the burn at the very least must involve the nerve plexuses conveying pain and therefore must be either deep dermal or whole thickness. The two advantages claimed by the proponents of tangential excision are:

1. If it is found that the subdermal veins are black in colour and obviously thrombosed the surgeon is immediately able to appreciate that the burn involves the whole thickness of the

skin and that excision must be carried deeper before the application of a graft.

2. If the reverse is the case and the burn is more superficial than expected no harm will come of the procedure because the whole purpose of tangential excision is to leave the deeper parts of the skin with its contained sweat ducts, and if the burn proves to be more superficial than the base of the hair follicles then healing will naturally occur within three weeks.

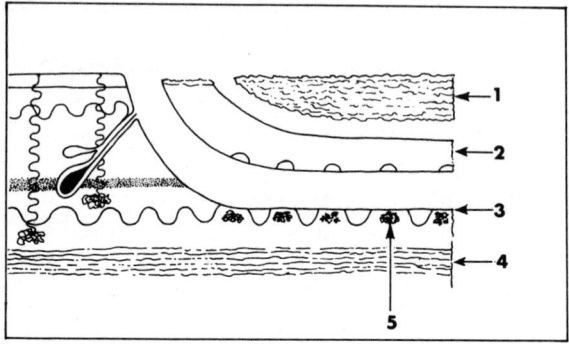

Fig 18.1 Schematic drawing to represent tangential excision for a deep dermal burn
1. First slice through burn
2. Second slice through burn
3. Base on which skin graft will be laid
4. Subdermal plexus remains intact, stasis but not thrombosis
5. Sweat gland remnants

Technique. The excision is performed between the second and fifth days following injury, having first eliminated *Streptococcus pyogenes* infection by the prior administration of an appropriate antibiotic such as erythromycin. The other serious infection with *Ps. aeruginosa* does not normally present a problem within the first week of burning.

The area of total anaesthesia is mapped out prior to the anaesthetic being administered and then, following anaesthesia, with a Braithwaite knife set to give a fine cut, tangential slices of skin are removed, starting from the centre of the burn which is most likely to be the deepest part of the burnt area.

As the slices reach the deeper parts of the dermis it will become obvious whether the subdermal plexus is thrombosed; if this proves to be the case the area should be excised with a scalpel until a suitable graft bed has been established.

When no thrombosed veins are visible and the tangential excision has reached the fat domes, or a little above, the case can be considered suitable for grafting. At this point, if the procedure has not been carried out under a tourniquet, the dermis will be pink in colour and mutiple bleeding points will be seen.

In this plane, if the burn is treated merely by dressing, further necrosis will occur whereas if the dressing used is a split thickness graft these will take. The punctuate haemorrhage which occurs should be controlled by the application of warm moist saline packs before the grafts are placed in position and because haematomata may develop, the area should be dressed on the second day and such haematomata evacuated. The extent of the area submitted to excision at any one time is determined by the availability of blood and donor skin since considerable bleeding may occur. The availability of donor skin is particularly important because the graft must be placed on the excised dermis at once, otherwise, if the area is left exposed, the residual dermis will slough.

The donor skin should be a thin razor graft (Fig. 18.2) and the grafts should be placed edge to edge leaving no intervening bare area.

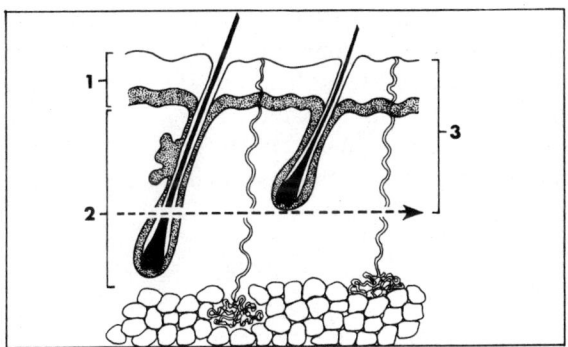

Fig 18.2   Split thickness graft suitable for a burn. Using this type of graft it should be possible to take a second graft in two to three weeks.
1. Epidermis
2. Dermis
3. Thickness of skin graft removed

A normal 'take' can be assumed if the grafts appear pink between the second and third day. If the graft fails it probably means that it has been put on a bed on which too much ischaemic dermis remains.

Following the completion of the operation a dressing is applied, the one described by Jackson being tulle gras soaked in neomycin and chlorhexidine, external to which a layer of cotton wool moistened in 0.5% silver nitrate, and finally, a crepe bandage.

COMPLICATIONS OF SEVERE BURNS OR SCALDS

Immediate complications

Infection

A burnt or scalded individual is in danger of developing a variety of infections including:

1. *Clostridium tetani.*
2. *The gas gangrene group of organisms.* Such infections may occur in a whole thickness burn involving muscle. Therefore until excision, prophylactic ampicillin and metronidazole should be administered.
3. *Streptococcus pyogenes.* This organism causes delayed wound healing, failure of skin grafts to take, and possibly septicaemia. *Strep. pyogenes* once represented a major problem but it has now lost much of its pathogenicity and the cessation of the routine prophylactic administration of antibiotic therapy at the Mount Vernon Burns Unit did not lead to any increase in complications from this organism. This group recommend that systematic antibiotics should only be given immediately prior to debridement. The antibiotic given being determined by preoperative wound cultures.
4. *Pseudomonas aeruginosa.* This organism colonizes the burn from the fifth day onwards. Clinically, the infection is recognized by the bluish green pus present on the dressings, and if there is a concommitant infection with *Ps. proteus* the pus will also be foul smelling. The use of silver sulphadiazine delays colonisation by these organisms and, therefore, reduces the danger of septicaemia. This would be recognized by the development of chills, hyperpyrexia or hyperthermia, tachycardia, tachypnoea, hypotension and the onset of oliguria.

A vaccine against *Pseudomonas* infection is undergoing trials at the present time.

All the hazards of infection are, of course, reduced by early excision and grafting or by tangential excision and grafting, whichever is appropriate, and they have also been reduced by the vast array of available antibiotics. However, the increasing use of antibiotics and the conquest of burn shock have led to fungal infections assuming an increasing importance in burns, the control of which is difficult.

Duodenal and gastric ulceration

This form of peptic ulceration is commonly referred to as Curling's ulcer. The incidence increases as the area of the burn increases, as demonstrated by routine fibre endoscopy in extensively burned patients. Fibre endoscopy has shown that a large percentage of patients in whom a 30% burn or greater has occurred develop acute erosions in both the stomach and the duodenum and that it is from these acute lesions that penetrating ulceration develops. The development of the latter appears, however, to be related to the pH of the gastric juice and it would seem reasonable to administer cimetidine to all extensive burns in the hope of aborting this complication which may lead to severe upper gastrointestinal bleeding.

Renal failure

Severe burns inadequately resuscitated may be followed by either oliguric or less commonly non-oliguric renal failure.

Liver necrosis

A complication usually following prolonged untreated shock, the typical lesion is a centrilobular haemorrhagic necrosis.

Pulmonary complications

1. Noxious combustion products might have been inhaled. Physical signs appear in the chest after 24–48 hours of injury and, at the same time, derangement in the blood gases develops. If death ensues, post mortem shows congestive oedema and sloughing of the bronchial mucosa.
2. Pulmonary oedema due to overloading of the circulation during resuscitation.
3. Pulmonary atelectasis due to excessive bronchial secretions.

Encephalopathy

In young children there may be a burn encephalopathy, due to cerebral oedema following resuscitation. Treatment by adrenergic blocking agents, e.g. chlorpromazine, and increased fluid intake and a heat cradle are required. The latter dilates cutaneous vessels and produces increased surface heat loss, so lowering the core temperature which is abnormally high in this condition.

Intermediate complications

1. *Pseudomonas aeruginosa* septicaemia.
2. Pneumonic lung changes.
3. Embolic lung phenomena.
4. Ducubitus ulcers. These are a hazard in any extensive burns and can be avoided only by frequent turning.
5. Constricting eschar. This may form if the whole circumference of the limb has been burnt or large areas of the chest wall are involved. The treatment consists of excising part or the whole of the constricting lesion.

Late complications

1. Contractures. Inevitable contractures follow burns of flexion surfaces or if loose ends such as the eyelid, ear, or lips are involved.
2. Hypertrophic scars. These are particularly liable to follow the spontaneous healing of the deep dermal burn which is one of the reasons for adopting tangential excision and grafting.
3. Pruritis. This is usually a self-limiting complaint but may be exceedingly troublesome.

19 Malnutrition and its treatment

Any patient in whom the normal requirements of calories, normally some 30–50 kcal/kg bodyweight per day, cannot be consumed has to draw on the body reserves. Normally, an individual requires between 2000 and 2500 kcal/day, but this may rise by some two and a half times in a patient who is, for example, suffering from severe burns.

A normal 70-kg man has a reserve of only 600 g of sugar, stored chiefly in the liver as glycogen, and this is rapidly exhausted.

The greatest store of calories in the body is fat, which provides 9 kcal/g, but whilst most tissues will accept fat as their source of energy, the central nervous system, the red cells and the renal medulla require sugar. Since fat cannot be converted to sugar, to supply these essential systems with energy the starving individual not only consumes his fat reserves but also breaks down some protein to convert to sugar by the process of gluconeogenesis. Thus sugar when administered as part of an elemental or parenteral diet acts as a 'protein sparer', but even in the presence of excessive sugar some protein breakdown still occurs and it is in order to diminish this that amino acids must be a part of such diets.

In total starvation, if an individual was able to survive by the breakdown of fat alone, some 200 g/day (each gram liberating 9 kcal) would provide the necessary energy requirements. However, since some 250–400 g of muscle (1 g of muscle yielding only 1 kcal) must be broken down daily to provide the 65–100 g of protein needed to provide sugar for those tissues which demand sugar as their source of energy, the total loss of weight per day may approach 1 kg or even more.

More important still is the fact that there are only 10 kg of protein in the body, only one half of which is in the muscles, and therefore the total lean body mass could in theory disappear in two months. Fortunately, adaptation takes place; the brain learns to use keto-acids derived from fatty acids so that the urine nitrogen loss of 10–15 g/day derived from the breakdown of 65–100 g of protein falls to between 3–4 g. Thus, the total bodyweight is reduced (although this may take some weeks to occur), by between 250–300 g/day of which only 10% is protein.

It is generally agreed that a weight loss of 10% of the total bodyweight at a rate of 300 g/day, which requires some three weeks, is tolerable, but that if this loss continues and reaches 33–50% death is almost inevitable, the protein loss rather than the fat being the most important factor.

WEIGHT LOSS

A simple clinical observation which gives some indication of weight loss is to examine the fit of an individual's clothes. More accurately, it can be quantified by a comparison between the present weight and the ideal weight derived from the height of the patient, remembering, however, that it is possible to be obese and malnourished at the same time. A patient consuming more calories than necessary adds to his or her muscle mass only if he or she exercises. In the absence of such exercise the extra calories are diverted into fat. The presence of oedema may also disguise the true state of affairs. The contribution made by fat and protein can be judged clinically by palpation of the subcutaneous tissues and the muscle bellies, loss of the former indicating fat loss, and loss of the latter, protein.

In the laboratory, protein turnover and lean body mass can be measured by estimating the 24-hour creatinine output in the urine, normally equal to the weight in kg × 23 in the male, or × 18 in the female. A patient who has lost only fat would have the expected creatinine output, as would anyone whose lean body mass is within normal limits.

A further parameter is the serum albumin: a value of 35 g/l or below indicates a severe problem, a value of the order of 25 g/l indicates a depletion of two-thirds of the total body albumin.

Other indicators of malnutrition are:

1. A profound fall in the lymphocyte count.
2. Immuno-incompetence as indicated by delayed hypersensitivity.

In general, operative morbidity and mortality are commonly increased when some 20% of the total bodyweight has been lost.

ENTERAL FEEDING

Indications

There are numerous indications for enteral feeding in the presence of malnutrition. These include leakage from oesophageal anastomoses, some gastrointestinal fistulae, inflammatory bowel disease, pancreatitis and colonic fistulae.

Methods

Gastric feeding

Gastric feeding is administered by means of a small-calibre, No 7 Fr gauge, flexible, silicone rubber tube with a weighted tip.

Jejunostomy feedings

This method is particularly useful when there is oesophageal obstruction or if a fistula develops after oesophageal resection.

A small incision is made in the upper abdomen and, having identified a loop of jejunum some 30 cm from the duodenojejunal flexure, a submucosal tunnel is created using a needle which will permit the passage of a long plastic catheter with an internal diameter of 1.0 mm. The catheter is threaded through the needle, which is then withdrawn. The point of entry through the wall of the gut is 'closed' by a purse-string suture, after which the needle is introduced through the abdominal parietes and the catheter brought to the surface. The jejunum is then stitched to the peritoneum and the abdominal wound closed.

The advantage of feeding by a tube resident in the stomach is the ease with which the method can be used. Its disadvantages are that an unconscious patient may regurgitate, and that in the conscious patient the appetite is 'killed' so that regular meals are no longer tolerated. The advantage of jejunal feeding is that the patient can still take food orally, but it has the disadvantages (1) that surgical intervention is necessary to insert the tube, and (2) that since the jejunum is sensitive to tonicity, intolerance and diarrhoea may follow unless time is taken to bring about tolerance. This is achieved by the use of low concentrations at first, followed by slowly increasing concentrations of the chosen enteral feed.

The overall benefit to the patient can be judged by an increase in well-being, in weight and in the plasma albumin.

A commonly used enteral feed is Vivonex (Norwich Eaton) which provides nitrogen in the form of pure amino acids, fat as highly purified safflower oil (80% as triglyceride of linoleic acid) and carbohydrate as glucose solids. The amino acids contribute approximately 8% of the calories, the fat 1.3% and the carbohydrate 90%. To each packet of 80 g is added 250 ml of water, 6 packets providing 1800 kcal/day, 5.88 g of available nitrogen, 2.61 g of fat and 414 g of carbohydrate plus vitamins and electrolytes. Alternatives are Clinifeed or Isocal.

PARENTERAL NUTRITION

Indications

As a general principle, parenteral nutrition is only necessary in that small group of patients whose metabolic needs cannot adequately be met via the gastrointestinal tract. Thus the chief indications for its use are:

1. Patients suffering from the short bowel syndrome as a result of massive resection. In this type of patient, intravenous feeding saves the patient from starvation during adaptation.
   Permanent parenteral nutrition has been adopted in a minority of patients suffering from this condition in certain specialized centres.
2. In patients in whom high-output enterocutaneous fistulae have followed surgery. Not only does parenteral feeding maintain the nutritional state of the patient, it also, in the absence of a specific disorder such as Crohn's disease, leads in a large proportion of cases to spontaneous closure of the fistula.
3. In patients suffering from severe trauma or sepsis in whom a hypercatabolic state with rapid weight loss occurs, e.g. severe burns, major sepsis or the complications of acute pancreatitis.
4. In patients suffering from Crohn's disease of the small bowel. There is some evidence that parenteral feeding may lead to remission.
5. Preoperatively in severely debilitated patients. There is some evidence that parenteral feeding administered over a period of 10–14 days prior to operation may reduce mortality. There is

no evidence that short-term therapy is of any benefit whatsoever. Equally, there is no evidence that parenteral nutrition speeds postoperative recovery following uncomplicated surgery, and in patients with a functioning gastrointestinal tract, diets administered by a fine-bore nasogastric tube or by fine needle jejunostomy are preferable to intravenous nutrition.

Method

All nutrient fluids must be prepared under strict aseptic precautions.

The nutrient

The first step in planning a parenteral nutrition regime is to assess the patient's total nitrogen, calorie and fluid needs. The patient's electrolyte requirements may be simultaneously incorporated or may be given separately. Normally, after adjustment, 3000 ml providing 3000 kcal of a glucose/amino acid solution can be tolerated daily and may well prove sufficient.

The administration of amino acids alone to redress a depletion of lean bodymass fails because the amino acids will be used as fuel and will not be incorporated into cells. For incorporation to occur, 100–250 calories must be provided for every 1 g of nitrogen, either as glucose or fat.

The principle carbohydrates used are glucose, fructose and sorbitol. If glucose is used, 500 ml of a 50% solution added to an 8% solution of amino acids provides 150 cal per 1 g of nitrogen and provides a total of 1000 kcal/l. One of the great disadvantages of a high concentration of glucose is that it must be given via a central vein. Furthermore, glucose is dependent on insulin for its utilization, and in conditions associated with stress a relative lack of insulin together with glucose intolerance may be found.

If high urinary losses of glucose are to be avoided, glucose should not be given more rapidly than 0.4 g/kg bodyweight per hour.

Nearly 20 proprietary amino acid preparations are available, all of which contain L-amino acids. The composition of the ideal mixture is disputed. Freamine is used in many centres, whilst others prefer Vamin; the latter corresponds most closely to egg protein standard, which is recognized as the ideal for oral feeding.

In the majority of amino acid solutions, e.g. Novoplex 1600, the necessary amino acids are provided. This solution contains: Na 100 mmol, K 80 mmol, PO_4 38 mmol, Mg 7.5 mmol and 400 g of glucose, providing an energy content of 1600 kcal/l. In a stable patient, the energy, nitrogen and electrolyte needs can be provided by the administration of 1 litre of Freamine or Novoplex 1600 and 500 ml of 20% glucose together with 500 ml of Intralipid on alternate days. The Intralipid is not mixed in the same bag.

So far as the amino acid content of parenteral fluid is concerned, it should be remembered that the amino acids fall into two groups: the so-called non-essential amino acids, which are continually being formed in the body by the amination of carbohydrate and fat residues; and the eight essential amino acids, which the body cannot synthesize and which must be provided.

Fat emulsions can be used as an alternative source of calories. The only available fat emulsion in the United Kingdom is Intralipid (KabiVitrum) which contains fractionated soya oil 10%, fractionated egg phospholipids 1.2%, and glycerol 2.2% in water, this emulsion being available in a 10 or 20% solution. One litre of Intralipid 20% provides 2000 kcal and has an osmolality of approximately 350 mosmol/kg of water. The glycerine is added to make the preparation isotonic. The great advantages of fat emulsions are that they can be administered via a peripheral vein, they have little or no osmotic activity and, after being rapidly metabolized, they leave no harmful by-products.

Sodium can be provided as NaCl or Na acetate, but never as Na bicarbonate since this will change the pH of the solution and precipitate everything. In general terms, the daily requirement of Na is within the range of 100–150 mmol/day. Potassium is needed in large amounts in the circumstances in which parenteral feeding is required, to ensure that adequate protein synthesis can occur. The normal intake of potassium is 80–100 mmol but more may be necessary in severely catabolic patients or in those losing potassium from a gastrointestinal fistula, although the hourly administration should not exceed 10 mmol. In addition, calcium, magnesium and phosphorus should be administered, giving 2.5 mmol Ca/1000 kcal, 4 mmol of Mg/1000 kcal and 10 mmol of phosphorus as HPO_4/1000 kcal, again remembering that none should be added to the preparation in quantities liable to cause precipitation. As in any starving or hypercatabolic patient, both vitamins and trace elements must also be added.

When using an amino acid/carbohydrate preparation, a period of

3–4 days should be allowed for the patient to develop tolerance, particularly in regard to the increased output of insulin required to deal with the carbohydrate load. The solution should be given at a regular rate and the volume increased to between 3500 and 4000 ml if necessary to achieve a positive nitrogen balance and weight gain. A maximum weight gain of some 0.3 kg a day may be achieved; gains greater than this are usually due to fluid retention and should be avoided.

Administration

When fat emulsions, which are isotonic, are used as the principle calorie source, it is possible to feed many patients via a peripheral vein; the lower concentration of glucose then used leads to a reduced incidence of peripheral phlebitis, particularly if 1500 units of heparin and 15 mg of hydrocortisone are administered daily through the same line.

If glucose is the chief source of calories, the nutrient must be administered via a central vein. This should not be used for any other purpose. The site of entry should be occluded with a waterproof dressing which should be changed every 48–72 hours. The administration set should be changed every 24 hours. No additions should be made once the solutions have left the pharmacy.

The central catheter can be introduced into the superior vena cava via the subclavian vein by using the following technique. The patient lies supine on a firm bed with the foot of the bed slightly elevated. A small pad is placed under the upper thoracic spine to allow the shoulders to drop backwards. After preparing the skin of the neck, the skin, subcutaneous tissues and the periosteum of the under surface of the right clavicle just lateral to the midline are infiltrated with local anaesthetic. A 14-gauge needle, 5 cm in length, attached to a small syringe is then inserted through the skin and advanced towards a finger placed into the suprasternal notch. A rush of blood into the syringe marks entry into the subclavian vein, at which point the syringe is removed taking care to occlude the needle. A 16-gauge radio-opaque silicone catheter is then passed through the needle and threaded into the superior vena cava. The needle is withdrawn, and the necessary connection made with an intravenous administration set through which an infusion of normal saline is commenced. A dressing is applied to the insertion site after first anchoring the catheter to the skin by a stitch. A radiograph of the chest is taken at the end of the procedure to exclude a pneumothorax.

Monitoring

Careful biochemical monitoring is required, particularly in regard to:

1. Urine sugar. Overenthusiastic administration of carbohydrate may lead to an increase in urine sugar and an unwelcome osmotic diuresis. A constant glycosuria in a non-diabetic patient is an indication to slow the rate of administration or, alternatively, to administer insulin.
2. Calcium, since if phosporus is given in the absence of a sufficient intake of calcium, severe hypocalcaemia may develop. Conversely, if there is an inadequate intake of phosphorus leading to hypophosphataemia, a hypercalcaemia may develop.
3. Sodium, potassium and urea levels should be estimated daily, together with the haematocrit. With these values to hand, the following 24-hour treatment can be prescribed.
4. Zinc and magnesium concentrations should be estimated weekly, since it is difficult if not impossible to recognize a deficiency of these cations.
5. Accurate fluid balance charts are essential, and care should be taken to measure and chart all fistula and other gastrointestinal losses. Daily weighing is an invaluable aid to the assessment of fluid balance, an abnormal gain in weight usually reflecting fluid retention.
6. Liver function tests should be performed twice weekly because abnormalities of liver function are common during total parenteral nutrition.
7. The temperature, pulse and respiration rate should be recorded every six hours. If a sudden rise in temperature occurs, it must be considered to be due to catheter fever until proved otherwise. This occurs in a considerable number of patients, particularly if the precautions already described are not taken, and in some series published in the United States has accounted for a mortality of 2%. If fever does develop, blood for culture should be taken, the catheter removed over a guide wire, leaving this in place, and the tip sent for culture. The disappearance of the fever confirms the diagnosis of

catheter sepsis, and after 24 hours a new cannula can be inserted along the guide wire. Should the fever not abate, the guide wire should also be removed so that the patient can be observed without the presence of any foreign material to 'fog' the issue.

20 The relief of pain

THE ANATOMY OF PAIN

'Free' terminals are the only sensory endings sufficiently widely distributed to serve the almost ubiquitous sensitivity to pain. In some parts of the body, e.g. the cornea, they are the only form of innervation, and elsewhere they are distributed in varying density. The nerve fibres associated with pain are mostly relatively small and slowly conducting. Electrical stimulation of the sural nerve in conscious patients shows that pain is not produced until the smallest myelinated fibres are activated, and only becomes unbearable when unmyelinated fibres are aroused. As nerve fibres travel peripherally so they branch repeatedly, each daughter axon being smaller than its parent so that it is possible that some small unmyelinated fibres in the cutaneous plexus may be derived from large myelinated fibres in a nerve trunk. The unmyelinated fibres are four times more numerous in a cutaneous nerve than those which are myelinated, and in nerves supplying viscera this disproportion is even greater. The finely myelinated A fibres subserve unipolar receptors, and the unmyelinated C fibres, polymodal receptors. If a noxious stimulus is powerful enough, it will recruit fibres which normally carry other modalities of sensation. The A fibres are relatively rapid transmitters and, when stimulated, give rise almost immediately to a sharp pain; whereas the unmyelinated C fibres are slow transmitters producing a sensation of a duller more prolonged pain. In the skin of the human palm, the area supplied by a single myelinated nerve may vary between 10 and 600 mm^2, but such is the overlapping nerve network at the dermo-epithelial junction that even the finest natural stimulus inevitably arouses several fibres.

It was once believed that all the sensory fibres from the whole body, including the viscera, reached the central nervous system through the dorsal nerve roots or in the sensory root of the trigeminal nerve. Recently, however, it has been shown that nearly one-third of the ventral root fibres are unmyelinated and that approximately one-half of these are C fibres coming from polymodal receptors which respond to noxious or deep stimuli.

Visceral afferents run centrally along the same paths as the motor fibres of the sympathetic and pass through the sympathetic chain, although there is no essential difference, either anatomical or physiological, between the visceral and the cutaneous afferents.

When the peripheral nerves enter the posterior horn of the spinal cord, they divide into short ascending and descending branches known as the tracts of Lissauer and synapse with the second order neurones. This area has now been stratified into seven zones: an outer superficial zone and six deeper laminae. Each lamina receives its own direct input, although indirect stimuli may be received from an adjacent lamina so long as the input stimulus is above a certain threshold. The marginal lamina together with laminae LI, II and III and the substantia gelatinosa, receive both A and C fibres; laminae IV and VI, collectively known as the nucleus proprius, receive A fibres originating from pinprick receptors and thermoreceptors. Other receptor areas are laminae VII and VIII, the latter being situated within the anterior horn. Within the spinal cord there are two spinal pathways of pain perception: the short fibre or multisynaptic system; and the long fibre or oligosynaptic system.

The multisynaptic system is composed of the spinal reticular core together with Lissauer's tracts. Both these components lack somatotopic organization and passage of information to supraspinal levels is relatively slow. The oligosynaptic system consists of the exteroceptive fibre columns of the dorsal tract and the spinothalamic tract. Both are rapidly conducting, and both carry precise information and accurate localization of nociceptor stimuli.

The two systems are intermingled in the spinal cord but are separate and independent. The fibres of the spinothalamic tract relay in the ventrobasal thalamus and are then projected somatotopically to the postcentral gyrus and the sensory cortex. The cortex is intimately concerned with pain sensation and cutaneous pain can be localized with extreme accuracy; this is in contrast to visceral pain which is usually diffuse, possibly because the innervation of viscera is less overlapping than that of skin and therefore provides less information to the brain.

The spinoreticular system relays in the reticular system and is then projected to the intralaminar thalamus, the hypothalamus and the limbic system. Whereas the oligosynaptic system localizes the site of pain, the multisynaptic system underlines the diffuse, persistent quality of the fully appreciated pain. Each relay allows inhibition and summation to occur.

THE PHYSIOLOGY OF PAIN

Many investigators believe that every kind of trauma acts in the same way, by liberating a chemical intermediary, an algogen, from the damaged cells. Likely substances include histamine, bradykinin, leukotrienes and serotonin, all of which arouse pain when injected into the skin. Prostaglandin E, which is synthesized locally in response to very slight trauma, may be a precursor, since in the human it has been shown that PGE 1 lowers the threshold to chemical and mechanical stimulation and also induces hyperalgesia, possible by sensitizing the receptors.

It may be that pain production is normally modified by the intermittent formation and removal of one or other of these algogens in a fashion similar to the transmission of nerve impulses by acetylcholine at the synaptic junctions. In an inflammatory process many possible algogenic agents are liberated by tissue breakdown, and it might be that the non-steroidal anti-inflammatory agents relieve pain by suppressing the generation of algogens.

Whatever the nature of the most peripheral stimulus to pain production, neural transmission must bring the impulse to the first synapse and the second order neurone. At this point, summation of stimuli occurs or, alternatively, impulses descending from the brain lead to total suppression.

It has been suggested that onward transmission may be inhibited by the endogenous opiates. These are the enkaphalins and endomorphin. These chemicals are thought to bind to the opiate receptors on the nerve ends thus blocking the onward transmission of impulses to higher centres.

The enkephalins, met-enkephalin and leu-enkephalin have been indentified in the periaqueductal system, the substantia gelatinosa, thalamus, hypothalamus and the mid-brain, whereas β-endomorphin, which is a much more stable and potent compound, is found only in the hypothalamus and hypophysis. Both the enkephalins and endomorphin are released in the experimental animal by direct stimulation of the periaqueductal grey matter and by nerve stimulation, and their activity is blocked by the narcotic antagonist, nalaxone.

In 1965, Melsack and Wall published their hypothesis, known as the gate theory, that the fast- and slow-conducting fibres in the peripheral nerves activate opposing mechanisms. These, together with the descending impulses, determine the amount of input transmitted from the peripheral fibres to the centre, and once the output from the second order cell rises above a given level, pain is produced.

When pain is of visceral origin there is often 'referred' pain, in which a sensation of pain and objective hyperaesthesia of the skin occurs in the territory of the spinal segments supplying the affected viscus. The explanation generally put forward to account for this phenomenon is that the input from the disordered viscus and the input from skin converge on the same second order neurones.

That cutaneous and visceral sensation are carried in the same second order neurones is suggested by fibre counts which show many more fibres in the input channels of the posterior roots than exist in the spinothalamic tracts. If visceral pain is transmitted in a second order neurone of its own, it is probably localized to the ventral midline, but visceral pain can be referred to a distant focus even after this area has been denervated.

PSYCHOLOGICAL ASPECTS OF PAIN

It has long been recognized that, regardless of the anatomical pathways and physiological mechanisms associated with pain, psychological factors are of great importance. Thus the central processing of the input from the nociceptors is modulated by a variety of factors, including fear, anxiety, depression and the previous experience of pain. The importance of an individual's response to pain is illustrated by comparing the analgesic requirements of battle casualties with the requirements of civilians suffering an injury. The former require less – they have suffered an honourable release from danger – whereas the latter require more – they have suffered an unpleasant interruption of their daily lives. It has also been found that the dose of postoperative analgesics can be considerably reduced if the effects of the operation are explained to the patient. The sudden crescendo-like pain, so typical of the acute abdomen, seldom responds to placebos. However, with pain of slow or gradual onset, a placebo is effective in one-third of patients. Just as the severity of pain is related to the psychological make-up of the patient, so pain may change the emotional state of the patient, leading to anxiety, depression or even aggression. Meisky states that patients suffering pain of physical origin become more disturbed than patients suffering from functional pain. It is because of the psychological consequences of pain that the tranquillizing and anti-depressive drugs may be useful in treatment. Patients in acute pain frequently feel helpless, a feeling which enhances pain sensitivity. This feeling can be aided in a variety of ways: chiefly by cognitive control, in which the patient is asked to concentrate and re-interpret the pain sensation by denying its existence; or by behavioural control, using manoeuvres which decrease pain perception, such as breathing exercises.

MEASUREMENT OF THE SEVERITY OF PAIN

There is no scientific method by which the severity of pain can be measured. Several comparatively simple clinical methods are, however, available.

The simplest of these, in a cooperative patient, is the verbal rating scale (VRS) in which the observer merely notes how the victim classifies his pain, recorded simply as: none, mild, moderate or severe.

A slightly more accurate method, which demands greater cooperation on the part of the patient, is the Visual Analogue Scale (VAS) in which, using most commonly a 10-cm scale, the patient marks the intensity of his or her pain at intervals moving from the left of the scale, 'no pain at all' to the extreme right,' worst pain imaginable'. To compare the effect of different therapeutic methods, the pain intensity difference (PID) score can be used. In this, the intensity of the pain is recorded prior to, and at a given interval after, the administration of an analgesic or, possibly, a placebo.

TREATMENT

Pain may be treated in a variety of ways. The surgeon dealing with an acute abdominal emergency, severe trauma or postoperative pain, all of which are of short duration, attempts to relieve the pain as soon as possible by the use of narcotics. When the pain is chronic, especially if the cause is untreatable, a distinction must be drawn between those patients with a short, and those with a normal life expectancy.

In some patients, destructive neurosurgical procedures offer the best chance of relief. However, many of these have a high failure rate, with the return of pain following temporary relief which may be measured in months rather than years.

Pain-relieving agents are commonly divided into (1) those of mild or intermediate potency, and (2) the narcotic group, which may be subdivided in turn into naturally occurring and synthetic.

Mild analgesics

The non-narcotic analgesics probably block pain at the periphery. This group includes aspirin, which was originally developed as an anti-pyretic when it was noted that moderate pain could be relieved by its use. Aspirin is not very effective for the relief of visceral pain and is therefore not commonly used by the surgeon, but it is extremely useful to the orthopaedic surgeon. It may, however, produce significant morbidity, since gastrointestinal haemorrhage may follow its administration even when it is used in a soluble form to promote rapid absorption and thus rapid relief of pain.

If aspirin is combined with phenacetin and codeine a synergistic effect occurs, but the use of phenacetin may lead to papillary necrosis of the kidney with subsequent renal impairment. If large and repeated doses of aspirin are given, dizziness, tinnitus, sweating, nausea and vomiting may occur.

Paracetamol (dose 0.5–1 g) is the active metabolite of phenacetin and has a somewhat similar potency to aspirin but lacks the gastrointestinal side effects. Occasionally, patients manifest an idiosyncrasy to this drug and develop skin eruptions, urticaria or fever. The mean red cell life is reduced, an effect of little importance in adults but children under three months of age are particularly susceptible and should not be given this compound. Toxic doses of paracetamol vary according to whether large doses are taken over long periods, e.g. 5 g daily, or in a single dose; symptoms and signs develop in the majority of patients ingesting 15 g in a single dose. The symptoms of overdose include nausea, vomiting and abdominal pain, followed by jaundice 2–6 days later as hepatic necrosis develops. Any patient who has taken 7.5 g or more in a single dose should be regarded as susceptible to liver damage, and if seen within 10 hours the specific antidote, acetylcysteine should be given by intravenous infusion in an initial dose of 150 mg/kg bodyweight over 15 minutes, followed by 50 mg/kg over 4 hours, and then 100 mg/kg over the next 16 hours. Alternatively, methionine 2.5 g may be given by mouth every 4 hours for 16 hours.

Analgesics of intermediate potency

The chief member of this group is the drug, codeine, (dose 10–60 mg), which is a methyl derivative of morphia. Even in very large doses this drug does not produce central depression. When used to suppress pain, if the larger dose of 60 mg is not effective even larger doses will also fail and may produce restlessness and excitement.

Many combinations of codeine, usually with paracetamol, have been formulated by pharmaceutical companies. Many of these contain too little codeine to be really effective, but the drug marketed under the trade name of Tylex, containing 30 mg codeine and 600 mg paracetamol, is an effective combination in such conditions as acute back pain.

Other members of this group include dextropropoxyphene, an analgesic chemically related to methadone. This drug is also commonly used in combination with paracetamol, a popular combination being marketed under the name of Distalgesic of which each tablet contains 32.5 mg dextropropoxiphene and 325 mg paracetamol.

Potent analgesics

The 'gold standard' against which all other narcotic analgesics must be measured is the naturally occurring narcotic morphine. It was not until 1971 that the existence of the opioid receptors was discovered, and in due course it was established that the receptor system was composed of several distinct subgroups and a wide range of endogenous ligands. Three receptor groups – mu, kappa and sigma – were originally defined and more recently two further receptors have been discovered, the delta and the epsilon.

Drugs may act as agonists, partial agonists or antagonists at any or all of these receptors. An opiate, either natural or synthetic, acting on the mu(μ) receptor produces analgesia, respiratory depression, euphoria and miosis; one acting on the kappa receptor produces analgesia and respiratory depression, but the behavioural pattern becomes one of sedation; and with an opiate acting on the sigma receptor no analgesic effect is produced, respiration is stimulated, the behavioural pattern becomes one of dysphoria and the pupils dilate.

Morphia acts at the μ and kappa receptors but has no action on the sigma receptors. Buprenorphine, a synthetic opiate, acts as an agonist for the μ receptors but has no action on the kappa and sigma receptors; whilst nalaxone is an agonist against all three receptors and is thus used for the complete or partial reversal of opioid depression, including mild to severe respiratory depression induced by natural or synthetic opioids.

The different responses to various opioid drugs largely depends on their pharmacokinetic properties. Thus, morphine-induced analgesia occurs somewhat more slowly than that induced by the synthetic drug fentanyl because it is less soluble in lipids. Other factors, including liver disease and age, also exert their effects.

The list of natural and synthetic opioids is long, but most surgeons and anaesthetists use only the small selection with which they have become familiar. In dealing with postoperative pain, it is still standard practice in many hospitals to use the time-honoured prescription, p.r.n. giving the dose of analgesic on an 'as required basis'. However, many argue that this is highly inefficient, not least because the attendant nurses, having no personal experience of pain, cannot properly relate to their patients, and many now advocate other methods. One such is to maintain a steady state plasma concentration by patient-controlled analgesia (PCA). A continuous background infusion of the analgesic agent is delivered which is controlled by the carer, and on this the patient superimposes additional bolus doses. Such a method obviously demands reasonable patient cooperation.

A second approach has been the use of regional anaesthesia, the nerve block reducing the pain during operation and in the immediate early postoperative period prior to the systematically administered opioids becoming effective. This method is used in thoracic surgery in which only a unilateral approach to the cavity is required. If a local anaesthetic agent is injected at, or medial to, the posterior angle of the ribs, more than one thoracic nerve may be blocked as the solution spreads along the paravertebral space.

The adverse side effects of the opioid group of drugs even after normal doses are nausea, vomiting, constipation, drowsiness and confusion. Larger doses produce respiratory depression and hypotension, with circulatory failure, deepening coma and, finally, death. If toxic effects leading to more serious symptoms are present, the specific antagonist, nalaxone is used, giving doses of

44 mg intravenously, repeated at intervals of 2–3 minutes if necessary.

CHRONIC PAIN RELIEF

It is now generally accepted that psychological factors will act together with organic ones to generate or worsen the patient's perception of chronic pain. Many patients suffering from chronic pain exhibit the symptoms and signs of a depressive illness, whilst others may have a mental disorder secondary to their physical problem. Three modalities of treatment are therefore used in the treatment of chronic pain, frequently in combination: a psychological, a pharmacological and a physical approach.

Psychological treatment

The psychological approach to chronic pain may involve the use of drugs, since many of these patients suffer from varying degrees of anxiety or depression. In such patients there is therefore an indication to administer either a tranquillizing drug or an antidepressant as well as an analgesic.

The major tranquillizers include chlorpromazine 75–500 mg daily in divided doses, thioridazine 30–600 mg daily in divided doses, and trifluoperazine 2–30 mg daily in divided doses. All these agents may produce extrapyramidal effects in susceptible people. Chlorpromazine is typical of the major tranquillizers and causes drowsiness, dryness of the mouth, pallor, headache, fatigue and weakness. Jaundice may occur, usually within two weeks of commencing treatment.

The minor tranquillizers include the benzodiazepines, chlordiazepoxide 10–100 mg daily in divided doses, and diazepam 4–40 mg daily in divided doses, and the carbamates, of which meprobamate 0.4–1.2 g daily in divided doses is most commonly used. All these drugs may be used to suppress less severe degrees of anxiety but all tend to produce drowsiness.

The antidepressants are also divided into two major groups: (1) the direct antidepressants, of which amphetamine is an example, and (2) the indirect antidepressants, which are themselves divisible into the monoamine oxidase inhibitors and the tricyclic compounds. This second group contains the hydrazine derivatives, e.g. Nialamide and Phenelzine, and the non-hydrazine monoamine oxidase inhibitors, e.g. tranylcypromine sulphate.

The tricyclic antidepressants rarely produce stimulation or excitement, as may the monoamine oxides inhibitors, but they may cause sedation and anticholinergic effects. The toxic effects of this group include jaundice, restlessness, tremor, hypotension and palpitations. The hypertensive and the aged may suffer severe hypotensive effects. They should not be administered to patients suffering from glaucoma, should not be given for several weeks after coronary occlusion and should be used with care if there is a history of coronary insufficiency. The tricyclic antidepressants may require 2–3 weeks before a noticeable therapeutic effect is achieved. If a patient fails to respond to one drug, it is often beneficial to stop the drug and put the patient onto another member of the group. Commonly used members of this group are: imipramine hydrochloride 75–150 mg daily in divided doses; amytriptyline hydrochloride 75 mg, increasing to 150 mg in divided doses; and nortriptyline hydrochloride 20–100 mg daily.

In addition to or in place of these mood altering drugs, various forms of psychotherapy, operant conditioning and behavioural therapy have all been used, particularly in patients suffering from long-term chronic pain of non-malignant origin. Group behavioural therapy leading to more adaptive coping styles have become popular in the West but are expensive. The aim of such group therapy is to alleviate the sense of helplessness, the loss of self-esteem and the abrogation of personal responsibility which tend to afflict chronic pain sufferers, e.g. in chronic backache in which physical methods of treatment have failed. This group is by no means small. Some 30 000 of the total United Kingdom population are admitted to hospital yearly with backache, of whom 5000 eventually come to operation; of these, between 10 and 15% fail to be relieved of their symptoms.

Pharmacological treatment

The need for tranquillizers or antidepressants has already been described. The drugs used for the specific alleviation of pain include all the analgesics discussed above, together with the non-steroidal anti-inflammatory agents, such as indomethicin and ibuprofen. The use of this latter group of drugs remains empirical, but they may be effective in chronic pain-producing conditions such as degenerative disease of the skeleton. However, their administration is not without adverse effects, chiefly involving the upper gastrointestinal tract in which ulceration followed by haemorrhage may occur.

In malignant pain, the availability of morphine sulphate in a controlled release formulation, such as MST Continus (Napp), has profoundly altered and improved the quality of life in such patients, as also has the appreciation that two daily doses are not always sufficient to relieve such pain. A usual starting dose is 20 mg MST twice daily, with the patient being given the option of taking an additional dose (escape dose) if analgesia is inadequate. At the next assessment the escape dose is added to the total daily requirement and the 'by the clock' prescription increased accordingly. The initial nausea and drowsiness induced by such a regime normally disappears after three days, although the constipating effect continues. The same period is required to titrate the necessary dose, and if the initial dose is ineffective it should be increased by 50% immediately.

Endocrine therapy

In endocrine-dependent tumours, administration of the appropriate hormone may do much to lessen the chronic pain associated with skeletal metastases. Thus, the administration of oestrogens to a male suffering from skeletal metastases from a carcinoma of the prostate may help, and in a female suffering from metastatic breast cancer involving bone, medical ablation of the adrenal oestrogen may also be helpful, a technique which has now completely superceded surgical adrenalectomy.

Physical techniques

A variety of physical techniques are available to relieve chronic pain, the most aggressive of which is the destruction of nerve tissue by chemicals, by radiofrequency coagulation, by cryosurgery or by the actual division of nerve fibres.

Non-ablative methods

Non-ablative methods include acupuncture and electrical nerve stimulation.

Acupuncture. Despite extensive research, mostly conducted by the Chinese, a scientific basis for this modality of treatment has not yet been established. Various investigators have found that the prior injection of the opioid receptor blocking agent, naloxone, reverses the analgesic effect of acupuncture, thus suggesting a humoral mechanism. It is also interesting to note than the injection of a local anaesthetic into an acupuncture point abolishes the analgesic effect as well. There is no doubt that some patients benefit from such treatment, and the wise surgeon will do nothing to dissuade a desperate patient from consulting an expert in this field.

Electrical nerve stimulation. Electrical nerve stimulation can be achieved either transcutaneously, when the electrodes made of carbon-rubber are merely placed on the surface of the skin (TENS), or the electrodes can be implanted into the posterior extradural space. The pulse frequency, pulse duration and total duration of the stimulation can be controlled by the patient. The frequency can normally be varied between 15 and 299 Hz, the pulse duration between 50 and 500 µs and the output is normally adjustable up to 50 mA. Usually, a constant current is used with an impedance of 0–1000 Ω.

The suggested physiological explanation of the efficacy of this treatment is that stimulation of the dorsal columns produces a descending inhibitory stimulus to the posterior horn cells, and hence analgesia. The overall efficacy of this method is said to be low, but the author himself has used it to great effect following a crush fracture of three thoracic vertebrae. It has also been used to treat the intractable pain which follows avulsion fractures of the brachial plexus, and the pain associated with a phantom limb. The former often causes a constant pain of burning quality together with an intermittent pain of great intensity which lasts for only a few seconds. If this method is used in this condition, the electrodes must be placed proximal to the most proximal point of the anaesthetic area. In treating phantom limb pain, not only has cutaneous stimulation been used but also thalamic implantation of the electrodes.

Destructive lesioning

1. The thermal coagulation or ablation of dorsal root ganglia or, in the case of trigeminal neuralgia, the Gasserian ganglion, has been applied to the treatment of chronic pain, as also has division of the spinothalamic tracts.
2. *Destruction of the coelic plexus*, usually by alcohol or phenol has also been used for the treatment of intractable pain arising from such conditions as pancreatic malignancy.

3. *Percutaneous cervical cordotomy*. This operation was first
   described by Mullan. It is applicable to pain within the
   distribution of C5 to S5. The technique does not require
   general anaesthesia, but the patient must be very cooperative.
   The principles of the operation are as follows: A needle is
   inserted just below and behind the mastoid process and its
   position in the subarachnoid space relative to the dentate
   ligament is radiographically determined. Once it is thought
   that the correct position has been reached a trial stimulation is
   performed, the distribution of the subjective sensation
   indicating the probable distribution of pain relief following
   coagulative destruction.
4. *Leucotomy*. Although this operation is capable of reducing the
   affective element of pain it does not remove its perception.
   Furthermore, personality changes associated with this
   operation may be severe. It has therefore been replaced by
   operations on the limbic system, such as cingulotomy.

Unfortunately, in many patients in whom destructive lesions are
used to alleviate chronic non-malignant pain, e.g. the pain associated with avulsion of the brachial plexus, the operation may
produce only temporary relief, lasting perhaps 2–3 years before
returning.

21 Tissue transplantation

HISTORICAL BACKGROUND

In 1597, Tagliacozzi of Bologna wrote that the singular character of the individual dissuades us from attempting to transplant tissue from one individual to another, a statement which suggests that he himself had attempted such transplantation when reconstructing facial wounds. However, in 1906, despite this injunction, the first successful corneal grafts were being performed in humans although the underlying mechanisms responsible for their success were completely unknown. In 1902 Alexis Carrel perfected the techniques of vascular anastomosis and immediately showed that autografts were universally successful whereas allografts universally failed. These results were consistently repeated so that, as time passed, interest in transplantation was abandoned by practising surgeons.

However, transplantation remained of interest as a method of potential benefit in tumour research leading Schöne and others in the early 1910s, to discover the following facts:

1. That xenografts always failed.
2. That allografts usually failed although a primary 'take' occurred prior to rejection.
3. That following the rejection of the first graft a further graft underwent accelerated rejection, the so-called 'second set' phenomenon.
4. That the closer the 'blood relationship' between the donor and the recipient the more likely was a successful graft.
5. That autografts were always successful.

Because skin had been used by him as a control, Schöne also demonstrated that these findings relating to tumour transplantation were also applicable to other tissues. More interesting still, he observed that skin grafts failed more consistently than grafts of organs such as the kidney.

By 1916, Tyzzer had discovered that previous exposure to living cells was necessary to provoke a 'second set' response, that the predominant cell at the site of rejection was the lymphocyte and that immunity to foreign tissue was not inherited as a single Mendelian factor but depended on a complex of independently inherited factors.

In 1926, Murphy demonstrated the phenomenon of immuno-logical tolerance when he showed that a tumour grafted into a chick embryo enjoyed uninhibited growth until the 18th day of embryonic life at which point it underwent spontaneous rejection. He also provided evidence of the importance of the lymphocyte by demonstrating that the production of a lymphopenia inhibited graft rejection.

In the early 1930s, George D. Snell developed congenic mouse strains so carefully selected that they differed at only a single locus from their congenic cousins. Using this model he was able to demonstrate a locus intimately related to the rejection of tissue grafts which he labelled H (for histocompatibility). Immediately prior to the onset of World War II, Gorer discovered a haemoagglutinating antibody associated with the rejection of homografts, which appeared to suggest that the long-sought-after cytotoxic antibody responsible for tissue rejection might be associated with the blood groups previously discovered by Landsteiner.

Interest in transplantation now appeared to wane. It had provided no answers of practical use to oncologists and had so far had little influence on surgeons, apart from the opthalmologists who continued to transplant the cornea but without any under-standing of the scientific basis for their success. However, the onset of World War II, accompanied as it was by a massive increase in the number of burns suffered by both the civilian population and the armed forces, served to renew interest in transplantation, particularly in the problems associated with skin grafting. Medawar began to work on the problem, first in the human and later in the rabbit. Rediscovering and re-exploring the work of Schöne (1912), Tyzzer (1916) and Waglam (1929), Medawar concluded (1) that whilst he was unable to explain the significance of the lymphocyte, it undoubtedly took the place of the polymor-phonuclear leucocyte in the inflammatory reaction provoked by a skin graft and (2) that rejection could be modified but not completely blocked by treating the recipient animal with either nitrogen mustard or corticosteroids.

Later work showed that grafts implanted within cell-impermeable chambers evaded rejection even in a previously sensitized host, but that if lymph node cells were included within the chamber rejection proceeded normally. Slowly it became evident that skin, because of its rich vascular bed and direct access to lymphatic channels, was highly immunogenic, and equally highly susceptible to invasion by those effector cells responsible for rejection. The heart and lungs, on the other hand, connected to the host by only a few major blood vessels, were in part isolated from the immune response of the host. The validity of this interpretation was confirmed by the work of Billingham, who showed that even a skin graft could enjoy prolonged survival if it was transplanted into a raised dermal pedicle connected to the host only by an artery and vein and not by lymphatic channels.

Further immunological research now led to the discovery of the major histocompatibility complex (MHC) which is located in man on the short arm of chromosome 6. Since the human histocompatibility antigens were initially identified on lymphocytes, the human MHC-encoded proteins are known as human lymphocyte antigens (HLA). These major transplantation antigens can cause vigorous rejection within 9–12 days of a transplant. Other, minor histocompatibility antigens are encoded at general sites other than the MHC. In the absence of immunosuppression, they cause a less vigorous response, taking as many as 300 days to bring about the complete rejection of a homograft. However, such minor histocompatibility antigens cannot be dismissed since they can be highly immunostimulatory in individuals who have been presensitized to them by prior transplantation or transfusion.

PRACTICAL CONSIDERATIONS

Transplantation began to play a significant role in the treatment of disease in the early 1960s when following the development of adequate immunosuppressive techniques, it was introduced for the treatment of patients suffering from end stage renal failure. In addition to immunosuppression, increasingly sophisticated tests of compatibility between donor and recipient became available, and kidney preservation techniques were developed which meant that 'matched' donor kidneys need not necessarily be used on site. Each of these features will now be considered.

Donor preservation

Preservation following removal of the donor kidney from a 'brain dead' individual can adequately be achieved over a 24 hour period by packing the organ in an iced container after first perfusing it via the renal artery with a solution resembling intracellular fluid, such as Collins solution. If preservation beyond this period is required the technique of cold pulsatile perfusion is used which enables preservation of the kidney for about 72 hours. This latter technique is associated with a lower incidence of delayed graft function, but is more expensive and may be rendered useless by mechanical failure of the perfusing device.

Tests of compatibility

Prior to the introduction of the agent cyclosporine A, attempts were made to match carefully donor with recipient. This was performed initially by taking account of the most important genetic difference as expressed by the normal blood group antigens, a Group A recipient requiring a Group A or O donor and a Group O recipient a Group O donor. Later, attention was paid to the more minor blood groups P, M and N and, lastly, the HLA loci, particularly to the Class I MHC loci known as HLA-A and HLA-B and to the Class II encoded protein, HLA-DR. However, with the introduction of cyclosporine many centres have shown that close attention to matching conveys little benefit.

Technique

The technique of kidney transplantation is now fairly standardized. The extraperitoneal approach is used. A lower quadrant incision is made and the iliac vessels exposed. The renal artery of the donor is anastomosed end-to-end with the internal iliac artery of the recipient, or end-to-side with the external iliac artery. The latter is now being preferred because of the propensity of the internal iliac artery to develop atherosclerotic changes distal to its origin from the common iliac artery.

The renal vein is similarly sutured end-to-side with the external iliac vein. The ureter can be dealt with by performing a standard Leadbetter-Politano ureteroneocystostomy. This requires an anterior cystotomy and the creation of a posterolateral submucosal tunnel. The ureter is passed through the tunnel, spatulated and anastomosed in a mucosa-to-mucosa fashion to the bladder. The anterior cystostomy is then closed in two layers. The major difficulties encountered may be the presence of 2 or 3 renal arteries, which may involve suture of an aortic button to the side of the common or external iliac artery.

Surgical complications

These include:

1. Renal artery thrombosis or later stenosis.
2. The development of a lymphocoele resulting from the perivascular dissection and the increased flow of lymph associated with the presence of the graft. Such a collection may lead to ureteric obstruction and demand drainage.
3. Vesico-ureteric complications, including ureteric obstruction and the breakdown of the ureteroneocystostomy which is usually due to disruption of the distal ureteral blood supply during harvesting of the graft or its implantation.

IMMUNOSUPPRESSION

1. *Reduction in circulating lymphocytes.* Early efforts to delay the rejection of homografts involved attempts to reduce the number of circulating lymphocytes which could produce a host versus graft reaction. Methods of achieving this included:
   a. Whole body irradiation.
   b. The construction of thoracic duct fistulae.
   c. Antilymphocytic preparations prepared in horses and then refined to reduce or prevent heterologous protein reactions.
   d. Anti T-cell monoclonal antibodies.

2. *Donor-specific transfusions*, acting possibly by stimulating suppressor T-cells or by the production of suppressive anti-idiotypic antibodies.

3. *Corticosteroids.* The most effective of this group of drugs appears to be prednisolone. One of the primary actions of the steroids is to block the release of interleukin-1 by antigen-presenting cells but, in addition, within hours of an oral dose of prednisolone, a T-cell lymphopenia occurs due to margination of lymphoid cells from the recirculating lymphocyte pool into the lymphoid tissues. In all patients receiving a renal transplant, a small maintenance dose of prednisolone is given daily in combina-

tion with the immunosupressive drugs described below, and methylprednisolone in single large doses is commonly used to prevent rejection although some patients eventually develop 'steroid resistance'.

4a. *Azathioprine*. This drug is a derivative of 6-mercaptopurine and was the first immunosuppressive agent shown to be of great value following renal transplantation. Metabolized to 6-mercaptopurine it is incorporated into cellular DNA and inhibits the synthesis of RNA, thus accounting for its antiproliferative activity on the rapidly dividing activated lymphoid cell population with the result that blunting of the immunological response occurs.

4b. *Cyclosporine A*. Initially introduced as an antifungal agent, this drug was first used in the transplant field in 1979. Its primary action is to reduce the production of lymphokines, in particular interleukin-2 and gamma-interferon by activated T-cells.

The dangers associated with the sole use of this drug in high doses soon became apparent, in particular its nephrotoxicity and, even more serious, the development of lymphomata.

It is now common practice to maintain a transplant patient on a combination of azathioprine, prednisolone and cyclosporine A, a combination which has been shown to be synergistic.

GRAFT REJECTION

Hyperacute rejection

This type of rejection occurs within a few hours of the transplant being put in place. It is believed to be due to two factors: the cytotoxic T-lymphocytes and the action of lymphokines which, although not normally directly cytotoxic, regulate a wide variety of antigen-specific and non-specific immune responses by affecting the function of lymphocytes and other cells, particularly the macrophages.

Hyperacute rejection is avoided by performing a lymphocyte cross-match between any potential donor and recipient prior to transplantation. Lymph nodes from the donor are obtained when the kidney is removed, and preparations of single cell suspensions of donor T-and B-cells are made. To these suspensions are added recipient serum plus complement. If donor-specific lymphocyte toxic antibody is present in the recipient serum, this antibody will bind to the surface antigen on the donor lymphocytes, fix complement and lyse the cells.

Characteristically the kidney rapidly assumes a mottled cyanotic appearance. Pathologically, within minutes of vascularization leucostasis appears in the glomerular and peritubular capillaries followed soon afterwards by extensive microthrombosis and layering of the polymorphonuclear leucocytes on the vessels. Immunohistology reveals the deposition on the vessels of IgG, complement components and fibrin.

The treatment of this complication is the immediate removal of the kidney.

Accelerated rejection

This occurs when, after 2–5 days, renal function of the donor kidney rapidly deteriorates. Although it is an immunological response, control is difficult and if large doses of methylprednisolone bring no relief the kidney should be removed.

Acute rejection

This normally occurs one week to several months following transplantation, the majority occurring within the first six months and some three-quarters of these within the first three months. Acute rejection is associated with a deterioration of renal function accompanied by a rise in the blood urea and the serum creatinine. The clinical picture is variable. In an unmodified rejection the tissues surrounding the graft become tender, a mild pyrexia ensues and a moderate hypertension develops. This picture is now rarely seen and most patients remain asymptomatic even though renal dysfunction is occurring. Graft biopsy shows interstitial oedema and tubular destruction. The cellular infiltrate is composed chiefly of lymphocytes, some macrophages and a lesser percentage of plasma cells.

In addition to changes in the interstitial tissues, a perivascular round cell infiltrate is frequently present, together with a subintimal mononuclear infiltrate accompanied by varying degrees of endothelial cell swelling and intimal disruption of the vessels.

The histological picture is extremely important since in the presence of pure interstitial changes nearly 100% of the episodes can be successfully treated, whereas if the biopsy reveals vascular changes in either the small or medium-sized vessels the condition is much more serious.

Care must be taken in the interpretation of biopsies, since the interstitial mononuclear infiltration is not specific but may follow as a secondary effect of cyclosporine. Because of this lack of specificity, due weight must be given to the clinical picture and the biochemical findings when coming to a diagnosis and prognosis.

Treatment

There are two effective forms of therapy:

1. *High doses of steroids*, increasing the dose of prednisolone or infusing methylprednisolone. High doses of steroids block the acute inflammatory process and allow the cellular infiltrate to clear from the grafted kidney; they also prevent further infiltration, thus allowing renal function to improve.
2. *Antilymphocytic preparations*, including heterologous polyclonal antibodies directed at the T3 complex of the human T-lymphocyte. These agents act by removing the lymphoid population of the graft by coating the lymphocytes with the immunoglobulin preparation and allowing their removal from the graft with either sequestration or destruction in peripheral lymphoid tissue.

   In addition to the above specific effects on the target organ all produce a peripheral lymphopenia and a dramatic decrease in the circulating T-lymphocytes.

By the use of these methods some 90% of all acute rejection episodes can be controlled.

Chronic rejection

Chronic rejection occurs between 1 and 4 years in some 10–15% of transplanted cadaveric kidneys. The mechanism is unknown. Pathologically, the histological changes in the kidney resemble those found in chronic glomerulonephritis and, because the changes in the kidney principally involve the small blood vessels and are consistent with an intimal proliferative lesion, attempts have been made to control the condition by the use of the antiplatelet drugs, dipyridamole and aspirin. Other than by these agents, it may be possible to control the situation by increasing the dose of azathiprine or giving in addition a further immunosuppressive agent, such as cyclophosphamide.

Long-term results

The long-term survival of cadaveric kidneys using triple immunotherapy is now about 80% over five years, as compared to the situation prior to the introduction of cyclosporine A, when the five-year survival of kidneys taken from unrelated donors was only about 30%.

22 Biological aspects of tumour growth

INTRODUCTION

The overall size of a normal fully grown individual remains relatively constant. This does not mean that cellular division has ceased, although it is certainly true for the central nervous system which, once having reached maturity, slowly atrophies. This change is particularly evident in the basal ganglia where, if the atrophy is severe, it causes Parkinson's disease, and in the cerebrum, where it causes senile dementia. At the opposite end of the spectrum are the cells of the skin, the mucous membrane of the gastrointestinal tract and the haemopoietic system in all of which division occurs in order to replace effete cells. The rate of cellular division has been most throughly quantified in the haemopoietic system because the lifespan of an erythrocyte can be readily determined following labelling with radioactive chromium. Such methods show that the half-life of the erythrocyte is about 60 days and if the curve for loss of radioactivity is suitably corrected it is found to be almost linear, falling to zero in about 120 days. Since the average red cell count is 5×10^{12}/l and the average blood volume for a man of 70 kg bodyweight is 5 litres it can be calculated that the number of red cells replaced daily by the normal marrow is approximately 2×10^9. Despite this enormous number, control is maintained so that the count does not fall and lead to anaemia or rise to produce the equally undesirable condition of polycythaemia. Similarly, the time required for the turnover of the mucosal cells of the gastrointestinal tract has been established by the use of tritiated thymidine which is incorporated into the deoxyribonucleic acid of their nuclei, thus enabling the cells to be traced by serial biopsy. This type of investigation has shown that in the stomach and duodenum, the turnover time is approximately two days, in the jejunum four days, and in the rectum seven days.

The factors that control these normal processes of cell division remain uncertain, although it is relatively obvious that, ab initio, growth must depend upon some inherent property of the fertilized ovum. In the child, the presence of growth hormone is essential since it is responsible for the normal rate of protein synthesis and fat metabolism. Deficiency of growth hormone alone leads to one type of dwarfism, 'sexual ateliotic', in which the individual remains short but matures sexually. At the cellular level it has been shown that cells of like structure, e.g. embryonic kidney cells, aggregate together in tissue culture even though initially separated. Having come into contact with one another the ability of such cells to divide is limited, a limitation believed to be due to contact, one cell with another. Such contact inhibition can, however, be altered by treating the cell with proteolytic enzymes, and it has been assumed that this phenomenon must be absent in the malignant cell. The affinity of cells for their own kind must be of great importance in the development of multicellular animals but even so, not all groups of cells behave in the same manner; blood cells for example do not exhibit adhesiveness, nor to any great extent do malignant cells.

CELLULAR DIVISION

G_1 phase

The life cycle of a cell, whether benign or malignant, begins as mitosis is completed and the cell enters the G_1 phase, otherwise known as the interphase. The duration of the interphase varies greatly. In rapidly dividing cellular systems it is characteristically short, whereas in slowly proliferating cellular systems it is long. However, for all types of mammalian cell the length of the reproductive phase is relatively constant.

The reproductive phase can be divided into three parts during which different processes are presumed to occur.

S and G_2 phases

The S phase was identified during the 1950s, when isotope-labelled precursors of DNA became available, allowing recognition of the time taken for DNA synthesis to be achieved. Between the relatively long S phase and mitosis is a period, the G_2 phase, during which no as yet identifiable event is occurring.

Mitosis

Mitosis, was identified in the late 19th century, when stains were developed which led to the identification of chromatin. Four stages are recognized during mitosis:

1. The *prophase* during which the chromosomes become visible within the nucleus as long thin filaments which progressively shorten and thicken. At this stage each chromosome has already split into its two daughter chromosomes, the chromatids, although each pair is held together by the centromere. At the same time, the cytoplasmic body, known as the centriole, divides to produce two centrioles which move to opposite poles of the cell and it is from these bodies that the protein fibres known as the spindle radiate. As this phase ends, the nuclear membrane, which is composed of two laminae each about 7.5 nm in width, disappears.

2. The *metaphase*. During this phase the microtubules, known as the spindle, are formed and radiate from the centrioles situated at the opposite poles of the cell. The chromosomes arrange themselves in the equatorial plane of the cells lying across the developing spindle and attached to it by their centromeres forming the equatorial plate.

3. The *anaphase*. At this stage the two chromatids separate following a longitudinal division of the centromere. The spindle fibres now appear to contract, pulling the chromatids, which have become the chromosomes of the two daughter nuclei, towards the opposite poles of the cell. Once this has been accomplished a cleavage furrow appears in the cell membrane indicating the beginning of cellular division.

4. The *telophase* in which the chromosomes elongate and disappear as the new nuclear membrane forms and the spindle disappears. At this point cellular division is completed and the cell enters the resting phase during which the individual chromosomes cannot be detected inside the nucleus as discrete structures by a light microscope, although a few condensations of DNA can be recognized, one of which is the sex chromatin, the Barr body.

Thus, the sequence of steps during the life cycle of a cell capable of division is as follows:

a. G_1 (interphase), a prolonged phase during which unidentified processes are occurring.

b. S, during which DNA synthesis is occurring.
c. G_2, a short phase during which unidentified processes are again occurring.
d. M, mitosis.

However, it has been shown that some cells capable of division pass into a resting phase of variable duration known as the G_0 phase from which they may, following a suitable stimulus, once more pass into G_1 and proceed to divide.

The percentage of cells in the G_0 phase in the bone marrow has been variously estimated at between 20 and 50% of the whole cellular population. The common stimulus which promotes division of this particular cellular population is haemorrhage. The fraction of cells that are actively dividing, the growth fraction, varies in different tissues, but in 'tumours' it is estimated that as many as 90% of the total population of tumour cells may be in the G_0 phase. Further, in a malignant tumour the cell population is very heterogenous, consisting of some cells that are capable of an infinite number of divisions until death of the host occurs, and others that are capable of only four or five divisions before this particular 'clone' of cells dies out.

In vitro studies have shown that the various phases in the cell cycle vary a great deal in duration. The G_1 phase may last up to 30 hours, whereas the synthetic phase is normally between 6 and 8 hours, the G_2 phase between 2 and 4 hours, and mitosis is usually accomplished in 1 hour.

Biochemistry of cellular division

The two most important constituents of the cell with respect to cellular division, are the nucleic acids. These are made up of many thousands of units known as nucleotides, each of which consists of three further subunits, a phosphate group, a pentose sugar and a nitrogen-containing base. In DNA the sugar component is deoxyribose, whereas in RNA it is ribose.

DNA contains four different nitrogenous bases, the pyrimidines, cytosine, thymine and the purines, adenine and guanine. RNA also has four bases but thymine is replaced by a different pyrimidine, uracil.

The sugar and phosphate groups form alternate links in the chain and the nitrogenous bases are attached to the sugar units at right angles. The DNA complex exists as two chains which are twisted into a helix and wound around one another in a spiral fashion, the two opposing spirals being linked together by hydrogen bonds which connect the nitrogenous bases projecting into the space between the strands.

The nature of the hydrogen bonds joining these base pairs is highly specific so that adenine unites with thymine and guanine with cytosine. As a result of this arrangement, if the sequence of bases on one chain is known, those on the other can be deduced.

The structure of the DNA molecule ensures that when the cell divides, the sequence of bases which constitute the genetic code will be carried to the next generation so that the new chromosomes will be identical with the old. Replication or division of the RNA strand results from the breaking of the hydrogen bonds, which thus releases the base pairs. Such unpaired bases would be free to pick up other bases from their surroundings but, because of the specific nature of the hydrogen bonds, each can only join with one of the four available. Once the bases are paired, linking enzymes bring the sugar and phosphate groups together to form the new DNA strand.

CELL CYCLE OF THE MALIGNANT CELL

The word 'cancer' emotively suggests a mass of cells growing and spreading in a chaotic disorderly manner. However, this picture has been modified in recent years and it is now recognized that, whilst the manner in which a cancer grows differs from that of normal tissue, there is frequently a growth pattern which resembles that of the tissue of origin or at least of the embryonic germ layer from which both the normal tissue and the cancer is derived.

The cell cycle of a malignant cell is remarkably similar to that of a normal cell, the total duration varying between 40 and 80 hours. The reason a tumour grows is because any division of a cancerous cell increases the total cell population, whereas in normal tissue this only occurs when the individual is growing. Thus in normal adult tissues a cell divides only to replace a cell which has been lost.

The total increase in bulk, however, of a tumour system does not follow the pattern which would result from the repeated division of a single stem cell; if this were so the tumour would double with each succeeding cellular division. This is not so. Depending on the tissue studied, the doubling time of a tumour may vary between 4 and 500 days, being most rapid for the leukaemias and slowest for solid tumours.

This variation in doubling time is caused by a variety of factors:

1. Some cells in a tumour may not wholly escape host homeostatic control.
2. Whereas in normal tissues growth is regulated so that supporting vascular stroma grows and keeps pace with expanding cell numbers, this is not so in solid tumours. In the latter, vascular structures fail to keep pace with the growth of the tumour with the result that lack of oxygen may result either in actual necrosis of parts of the tumour or the cells become so hypoxic that they become quiescent. Experimentally it has been shown that the cell cycle time, i.e. the time required for division, remains the same in hypoxic conditions as in a well-oxygenated environment *but* the dividing fraction of cells gradually diminishes as anoxia becomes more profound.
3. Many tumour cells are so abnormal that they can divide only through a few generations before finally dying. Conversely the malignant transformation in some cancer cells may be so incomplete that they may even differentiate to function more or less normally.
4. Cell loss. Cellular loss from a tumour may be caused by a variety of factors:
   a. Hypoxia leading to an increase in the number of quiescent cells or actual necrosis.
   b. Physical loss of cells by either exfoliation, e.g. gastrointestinal and urothelial tumours, or by metastasization.
   c. Host resistance. The gradually increasing importance of cellular immunity in the host's defence against neoplastic cells is becoming increasingly recognized. It has been suggested that immunological surveillance by an immunologically competent host is capable of the total destruction of small tumours. It is also an undisputed fact that in patients in whom this system is damaged either by drugs, by radiotherapy, or as the result of immunodeficiency disease there is an increase in the incidence of tumours, particularly of the lymphoid system.
   d. Apopotosis. This phenomenon is observed in normal structures and can be defined as programmed cell death. It is the process whereby embryonic structures which do not

persist until adulthood are resorbed, e.g. the webbing between the fingers and toes of the human embryo.

Cell loss is a significant factor in the growth pattern of carcinomata and of less significance in sarcoma. In carcinomata it is estimated that about 70% of all cells produced are lost, whereas in sarcomata this figure is about 30%. However, it should be remembered that the size of an individual tumour depends not only on the cell loss factor but also on the number of cells dividing and the rate at which they are doing so.

It is chiefly the combination of these three factors which determines the doubling time of a tumour.

In human leukaemias, growth is exponential in that there is a proportional increase in tumour cells per unit of time, but this does not apply to the majority of solid tumours, which are those of greatest interest to the surgeon.

So far as the clinician is concerned, a cancer in a superficial organ such as the breast is rarely detected before it has doubled in size approximately 30 times, thereby producing a palpable mass approximately 1 cm in diameter and weighing between 1 and 2 g. The following 10–14 doublings, assuming uninterrupted growth is allowed to continue, will result in a mass approximately 1 kg in weight, by which time death has usually occurred. Obviously the duration of life is intimately related to the tissue within which the tumour is growing. A patient suffering from a carcinoma of the colon in whom hepatic metastases are already recognizable at the time of the initial operation may live for as long as three years, whereas the physiological consequences of increasing intracranial pressure produce death in a short time in patients suffering from primary or metastatic malignant disease of the brain.

INFLUENCE OF GROWTH PATTERN ON THE EFFECTS OF RADIOTHERAPY AND CHEMOTHERAPY

The effects of irradiation or chemotherapy on any given tumour depends upon a variety of factors:

1. The size of the growth fraction, since this fraction represents the most vulnerable cells.
2. The size of the quiescent cellular population, since this is composed of cells initially resistant but which may, following treatment, begin to proliferate.

3. The size of the cell loss factor. The larger this factor the more rapidly will the tumour become smaller.
4. Age of the tumour. In general, young tumours have larger proliferating compartments than old tumours, and carcinomata have larger proliferating compartments than sarcomata which tend to have large quiescent compartments. This may reflect the germ layer of origin of the two types of malignancy. Thus, tissues derived from ectoderm and endoderm have in normal tissues a high cell turnover and hence a large proliferative component, whereas tissues derived from mesoderm have little cell loss per unit of time.

23 Cytotoxic and hormonal agents: their effects on normal and tumour tissues

INTRODUCTION

An increasing number of cytotoxic agents have been discovered, most by chance, since the original observation that nitrogen mustard Mustine hydrochloride B.P. used in World War I as a toxic gas possessed antimitotic activity. The latest edition of Martindale lists over 60 cytotoxic agents in all, excluding chemicals such as tamoxifen, an anti-oestrogen, and aminoglutethimide which abolishes adrenal cortical secretion. The majority of cytotoxic drugs are not only antineoplastic agents but also immunosuppressants and because of their general effects upon all cells all are potentially potent poisons, many having a very small therapeutic ratio. The introduction of a cytotoxic agent into clinical practice follows three phases. In Phase I, the toxicity and clinical pharmacology of the drug is established; in Phase II, a study is performed to determine its efficacy in various types of tumour; and finally in Phase III, the effects of the drug are evaluated in greater detail before it is introduced into some combination.

CLASSIFICATION BY MODE OF ACTION

The mode of action of cytotoxic drugs can be classified in two ways:

1. According to the point in the cell cycle at which the drug exerts its effect. Thus agents can be divided into (1) cycle-specific or phase-specific drugs when they act only at a specific point in the cell cycle; and (2) cell cycle non-specific drugs which, although having no effect on resting cells in the Go phase, attack the cell at all other stages with the same degree of effectiveness. Examples of the former include

6-mercaptopurine, methotrexate and cytosine arabinase which act during DNA synthesis (the S phase), and vincristine and bleomycin which act only during mitosis. Examples of the latter group include cyclophosphamide, the nitrosoureas and adriamycin.
2. According to their pharmacological activity (see below).

1 Alkylating agents

The commonly used drugs in this group include thiotepa, phenyl-alanine mustard, chlorambucil, cyclophosphamide and bisulphan.

The alkylating agents cause the development of cross linkages between opposite guanine bases, thus binding the DNA strands together and preventing their replication. Any free guanine bases which remain combine with the agent used, thus preventing them from acting as templates for the formation of new DNA.

Other agents with an alkylating action include the nitrosoureas, carmustine and lomustine, streptozocin, cisplatin and procarbazine. Unlike many tumour agents, the nitrosoureas are lipid soluble and are, therefore, able to pass through the blood-brain barrier.

2 Antimetabolites

This group includes methotrexate, 5-mercaptopurine, 5-fluorouracil and cytarabine hydrochloride.

The action of the antimetabolites results from their structural similarity to the normal cellular metabolites required for protein synthesis, a similarity well illustrated by that which exists between methotrexate and the vitamin, folic acid.

Methotrexate is a folic acid antagonist because it has a much greater affinity for the enzyme dihydrofolate reductase than folic acid. Once methotrexate combines with this enzyme the combination is inseparable and as a result folinic acid, the essential coenzyme into which folic acid is converted, is no longer formed. In the absence of the co-enzyme the synthesis of purines and pyrimidines ceases. In a similar manner, 5-fluorouracil, which is a pyrimidine in which a fluorine atom is substituted for a hydrogen atom, probably blocks the enzyme thymidilate synthetase. This is essential to pyrimidine synthesis, deficiency inhibiting the formation of thymine and cytosine and so preventing DNA replication.

3 Vinca alkaloids

This group consists of vincristine and vinblastine. The vinca alkaloids arrest cell division at the metaphase by interfering with spindle formation so that the chromatids cannot be properly paired, and mitosis ceases.

4 Antimitotic antibiotics

In this rapidly expanding group is included compounds such as adriamycin, bleomycin, streptozotocin, actinomycin D and mitomycin C. These compounds exert their effect by forming irreversible complexes with single strands of DNA, inserting themselves between the bases and attaching themselves by hydrogen bonds to the guanine moiety of the DNA chain, thus preventing the synthesis of DNA.

5 Miscellaneous group

The miscellaneous cytotoxic drugs include procarbazine, hydroxy-carbamide, hexamethylmelanine and asparaginase. The latter compound is of particular interest because theoretically it exploits one of the few biochemical differences that exist between normal and malignant cells. Asparagine is an amino acid essential to human cells. Unlike normal cells, however, malignant cells are unable to synthesize it and as a result have to rely on the supply of this amino acid from the general pool.

Asparaginase is an enzyme that splits asparagine into aspartic acid and ammonia. Theoretically, therefore, if the body is flooded with this enzyme the body pool of free asparagine should fall and the malignant cell be denied an essential nutrient. Unfortunately, in practice the efficacy of this drug has not lived up to its theoretical promise. In a similar fashion, the drug phenylala-nine mustard has also been a disappointment. In theory, the latter drug should have been extremely effective in the treatment of malignant melanoma because melanin-producing cells require phenylalanine in order to produce pigment. Using phenylalanine mustard, therefore, it might have been expected that the alkylating agent would have been specifically taken into the melanoma cell in much higher concentration than into normal cells, thus producing differentially higher concentrations of the alkylating agent.

Whilst it is generally accepted that the effect of these various agents is mediated via their pharmacological activity, the proposition has been put forward that they may possibly act by altering the immunological status of the host. However, since all the agents are immunosuppressive, this appears unlikely.

EARLY TOXIC EFFECTS

Bone marrow depression

Bone marrow depression is common to all chemotherapeutic drugs, since the doubling time of the stem cells of the bone marrow is only 15–20 hours whereas in a tumour system the doubling time may be as long as 500 days.

White blood cells

The first noticeable effect is on the white cells, the life span of which is only 4–5 days. The normal white blood count is $4–11 \times 10^9/l$ and the absolute granulocyte count (total white blood cells (WBC) × percentage of granulocytes) is normally $2.8–7.0 \times 10^9/l$.

Granulocytopenia is defined as an absolute granulocyte count below $2.8 \times 10^9/l$. When the count falls to less than $1.5 \times 10^9/l$ the patient is at risk from infection, and below $1 \times 10^9/l$ infection, particularly by opportunistic or endogenous organisms, represents a serious threat.

If a granulocytopenia develops during the course of treatment, hospitalization should be avoided if possible as this only increases the risk of infection. The most important general measures which should be taken are strict aseptic techniques in handling an intravenous line, such as a Hickman catheter, and a high-protein, high-calorie diet. When overt infection occurs the patient, if hospitalized, should be isolated and broad-spectrum antibiotics administered.

White blood cell transfusions are possible after matching for ABO type and HLA (histocompatibility factors) as closely as possible. Donor white cells must be used within 24 hours. Characteristic reactions to WBC transfusion consist of fever, chills, headache, hypotension and vomiting. White cells have a short lifespan.

Platelets

Platelet depression may cause serious difficulty. The normal level is 140–440 000/µl, a risk of bleeding is present if the number falls below 50 000/µl and at 10 000/µl the risk is critical. The most dangerous spontaneous haemorrhage is into the central nervous system. In order to avoid bleeding, trauma should be avoided and care taken to be certain that drugs interfering with platelet function, such as aspirin, dipyridamole, indomethacin and anticoagulants, are not being administered.

Platelet transfusion is indicated at 1–5000/µl. Platelet concentrates containing 8×10^{11} viable cells can be obtained and repetetive transfusions may be necessary at frequent intervals. As the number of transfusions increases so does the likelihood of isoimmunization. Reactions during or soon after transfusion cause fever, chills, headache, flushing, nausea and vomiting. Platelet transfusions have to be administered via special donor sets incorporating filters to remove platelet aggregates which, if infused, are trapped in the pulmonary capillaries causing pulmonary oedema.

Erythrocytes

Anaemia of varying severity may develop, demanding the transfusion of compatible blood.

Nausea and vomiting

These are the commonest side effects of chemotherapy and are among the chief reasons for a patient refusing further treatment. The cause of these symptoms is stimulation of the chemoreceptor zone in the floor of the 4th ventricle, which then stimulates the vomiting centre in the reticular formation and increases vestibular sensitivity.

The immediate results of severe vomiting are dehydration, hypokalaemia and alkalosis, and repetitive vomiting may radically alter the nutritional status of the patient.

These side effects are particularly common following the administration of nitrogen mustard and cisplatin, but are relatively infrequent after giving chlorambucil and 6-mercaptopurine.

Control may be achieved by the use of non-oral antiemetics such as prochloroperazine or phenothiazine together with an antihistamine and sedation by the phenothiazines.

Alopecia

Cells in the hair follicles have a high metabolic and mitotic activity and are, therefore, highly susceptible to cytotoxic agents. Such materials affect either the hair roots, producing atrophy and rapid hair loss, or the hair shafts, producing patchy loss. The drugs particularly involved are bleomycin, 5-fluorouracil and vincristine. Two methods, neither completely satisfactory, of avoiding this complication have been developed, the scalp tourniquet and the ice turban. It is perhaps better to forewarn the patient and provide an adequate wig.

Damage to mucosal surfaces

This may produce a stomatitis and glossitis. Whilst in the gut mitosis ceases in the stem cells which lie in the crypts of Lieberkühn.

Stomatitis is treated with nystatin, and the diarrhoea of intestinal toxicity by adequate fluid and electrolyte therapy.

Extravasation at the time of injection

This may cause severe tissue irritation and possible sloughing. Two of the most irritating drugs are nitrogen mustard and carmustine.

LATE TOXIC EFFECTS

Certain conditions, e.g. acute lymphoblastic leukaemia in childhood and Hodgkin's disease in the adult, may now, after being successfully treated by cytotoxic agents, be followed by long-term survival. Thus, the longer term effects of these agents are slowly being appreciated. Considering individual drugs, it should be noted that, with the exception of methotrexate for the treatment of choriocarcinoma, no tumour is now treated by a single agent. All malignancies are subjected to combinations of drugs. The known long-term toxic effects of the various agents are as follows:

The alkylating agents

1. Chlorambucil: interstitial pulmonary fibrosis and an increased incidence of acute non-lymphocytic leukaemia in children treated with drug.

2. Cyclophosphamide: bladder cancer.
3. Phenylalanine: acute leukaemia.
4. Cisplatin: peripheral neuropathy and hearing loss.

The antimetabolites

1. 5-Fluorouracil: neurotoxicity causing cerebellar damage and cardiotoxicity.
2. 6-Mercaptopurine: hepatocellular damage.
3. Methotrexate: used as a single agent in the treatment of choriocarcinoma and psoriasis may cause some hepatic damage.

Vinca alkaloids

Vincristine and vinblastine both cause neurological damage resulting in peripheral neuropathy, paraesthesia, weakness and abdominal pain.

Antimitotic antibiotics

1. Adriamycin: cardiomyopathy occurs with high doses, in 3% of patients when the total dose is 450 mg/m^2, rising to 10% if the dose exceeds 700 mg/m^2.
2. Bleomycin: interstitial pulmonary fibrosis follows total doses in excess of 400 mg.

Non-specific complications

In addition to the above specific complications there is good evidence that many of the alkylating agents are carcinogenic in man, and animal studies strongly suggest that drugs such as cisplatin, the nitrosoureas and procarbazine will prove similarly dangerous.

So far as combination therapy is concerned there is no doubt that quadruple therapy for Hodgkin's disease is followed by an increased risk of malignancy, particularly of acute nonlymphocytic leukaemia in patients treated with the classical combination of mustine, vincristine, procarbazone and prednisone. This risk is particularly evident if the patient has also received irradiation as part of the therapeutic regime. Furthermore, the risk of developing solid tumours is relatively high, in one reported series 7.3%.

In childhood, the successful treatment of osseous, renal and a miscellaneous group of soft tissue tumours is followed by a higher than anticipated number of second primary tumours. An exception is acute lymphocytic leukaemia. Although the successful treatment of this condition may result in long-term effects in the hepatic, pulmonary and skeletal systems together with mental changes, it does not appear to be followed by a higher than average number of malignancies, possibly because the combination of drugs used, i.e. vincristine, methotrexate and mercaptopurine do not individually or collectively appear to be carcinogenic.

In addition to these common effects the surgeon should also remember:

1. That the embryo is a mass of rapidly dividing cells and that cytotoxic agents given in the first trimester are a potent cause of fetal abnormality.
2. That the lymphoid system, which is responsible for the production of the immunoglobulins and immunologically competent lymphocytes, may also be damaged. This has two possible adverse effects: first, a failure to form antibodies and, hence, an increased susceptibility to infection, a susceptibility increased by the concomitant decrease in the granulocyte population; and secondly, a potential loss of those immune mechanisms helping to suppress tumour growth.

EFFECT OF A CYTOTOXIC AGENT ON THE TUMOUR CELL

When initially introduced, single cytotoxic agents were most commonly used over long periods in doses that caused minimal signs of toxicity. This technique was in accord with the then accepted principle that tumours increased in size because their cell population divided more rapidly than those of normal tissues. Approximately 20 years ago, combination therapy was introduced in which two or more drugs, each with a different effect on the dividing cell, were used. This system had the advantage not only of making a 'two pronged' attack on the tumour itself, but also of reducing the overall toxicity of a cytotoxic schedule since advantage could be taken of the differences in toxicity that exist between the different groups of drugs.

A further advance was made when intermittent chemotherapeutic regimes were introduced. These were based on the work of

Howard Skinner in the United States, in 1964, who studied the effects of chemotherapy on mice injected with L1210 leukaemia cells. He showed:

1. That the percentage of a leukaemic cell population killed by a given dose of a drug was virtually constant and *not* a fixed number of cells.
2. That the proportion of cells killed is proportional to the dose, assuming a sensitive malignant cell population.
3. That the rate of replication of tumour cells appears to be fixed, so that after the death of a proportion of them, the growth rate of the remainder does not accelerate to make up for the deficiency, as with normal tissue cells.

This last finding is of great importance since it indicates that the continuous use of a cytotoxic agent does not make optimum use of its potential since the reduction of tumour mass, if the drug is given in tumouricidal doses, will eventually be accompanied by signs of toxicity which may necessitate the cessation of treatment. In theory, by intermittent therapy it should be possible to eradicate the tumour without causing too much damage to the body as a whole. However, the timing of such therapy is critically important; too short an interval between courses may result in evidence of systemic toxicity whereas too long an interval may allow the tumour to recover completely.

Intermittent therapy is now generally used in tumour therapy. Apart from reducing the overall toxicity of a chemotherapeutic programme, it allows higher individual doses of the appropriate agents to be given, thus increasing the proportion of cells killed with each course of treatment. However, despite the theoretical advantages of this type of therapy, the vast majority of tumours cannot be completely cured because:

1. The response of a tumour depends upon the growth fraction. Whereas in Skinner's experimental model the growth fraction was nearly 60%, it may be as low as 10% in solid tumours, and since chemotherapeutic agents can only act against dividing cells, the bulk of cells in the average solid tumour, excluding the lymphomata, are resistant.
   The small growth fraction in solid tumours is partially explained by the degree of hypoxia within the centre of the tumour. This leads to a diminished growth rate and also to poor penetration of the tumour by the agents used.

2. The effects of chemotherapy also depend upon the cell loss factor. A tumour with a large growth fraction and a high cell loss factor is much more vulnerable than a tumour with low growth fraction and small cell loss factor.

Since a clinically detectable tumour is a 'late' tumour, few can be cured. However, adjuvant therapy is increasingly favoured in patients from whom the primary tumour has been eliminated by surgery in an attempt to control occult metastases.

The proponents of adjuvant therapy point out that the optimum time to produce tumour kill is when the tumour cell population is small, a period usually associated with the highest growth fraction.

The arguments against adjuvant therapy are:

1. The difficulty of selection.
2. Many patients may be treated unnecessarily.
3. The long-term adverse effects of such treatment may be undersirable.

Table 23.1 lists tumours found to be potentially curable by the use of cytotoxic agents.

Table 23.1   Tumours potentially curable by cytotoxic agents

Tumours of the lymphoid system	Acute lymphocytic leukaemia in childhood
	Burkitt's lymphoma
	Hodgkin's lymphoma
	Non-Hodgkin's lymphoma
Tumours of soft tissues	Embryonal rhabdomyosarcoma of childhood
Tumours of bone	Ewing's sarcoma
Tumours of the renal tract	Wilm's tumour of childhood
Tumours of the genital tract	Gestational tumours
	Testicular tumours

Many other tumours may be partially controlled by the use of chemotherapeutic agents, when a subjective response to treatment may be obtained or a temporary arrest of tumour growth be achieved as, for example, in carcinoma of the breast or the lymphocytic and non-lymphocytic leukaemias of adult life.

HORMONAL TREATMENT OF MALIGNANT DISEASE

In addition to the cytotoxic agents, the sex hormones, steroids and antisteroid drugs have a place in cancer chemotherapy.

The oestrogens

The seminal work on the place of hormones in the treatment of cancer was performed by Charles Huggins of Chicago some 50 years ago when he demonstrated that some tumours of the prostate and breast were hormone dependent, and that orchidectomy in the male and oophorectomy in the female controlled at least temporarily a proportion of tumours occurring in these organs.

Such was the initial enthusiasm that at first all patients suffering from carcinoma of the prostate were subjected to orchidectomy followed by the daily administration of stilboestrol 10–20 mg orally.

This early uncritical use of oestrogen therapy in a predominantly ageing population was brought to a halt by the surveys conducted by the Veterans Administration Co-operative Urological Research Group. Between 1964 and 1971 they published a series of papers which indicated that treatment of the ageing male with oestrogens may be harmful rather than beneficial, predisposing this population to death from heart disease or pulmonary embolus. They concluded that the hormonal treatment of carcinoma of the prostate should be withheld until palliation was required; in other words, bone pain was occurring uncontrolled by other means.

Similarly, oestrogens and androgenic hormones and progestins have all been shown to exert a beneficial effect on a proportion of women suffering from breast cancer, particularly when the sufferer is postmenopausal. At the present time, adrenalectomy and oophorectomy which totally ablate oestrogen have been replaced by the administration of aminoglutethemide in patients suffering from disseminated disease. This drug inhibits adrenocortical steroid synthesis and thereby reduces the production of adrenocorticoid synthesis. A dose of 250 mg four times a day is required, giving hydrocortisone 20–25 mg to replace the absent glucocorticoids.

OTHER TREATMENTS

In recent years, the drug tamoxifen (developed by ICI) has been extensively used for the treatment of patients suffering from breast cancer in which lymph node biopsy has shown involvement of the axillary nodes. Its exact mode of action remains controversial. Controlled trials between 1977 and 1981 supported the view that the administration of tamoxifen following surgery and radiotherapy produced a prolongation of the disease-free interval without significantly decreasing the overall mortality. In the early trials, the menopausal status of the patient appeared to be unimportant, but more recently it has been shown that the highest response rate occurs in women more than five years' postmenopausal. As a result of its lesser side effects, tamoxifen has now replaced oestrogens as the treatment of choice in this group of women.

Other methods, all at present of only theoretical interest, by which it has been suggested that malignant disease could be controlled are:

1. By the development of drugs capable of affecting tumour angiogenesis.
2. By drugs which prevent cellular implantation upon which the successful development of metastases depends. To this end, heparin has been given to prevent metastases developing after excision of the primary tumour.
3. By the development of cytostatic agents capable of arresting cellular growth.
4. By increasing the specificity of the agent.

24 Radiotherapy and malignant disease

Radiotherapy is the application of ionizing irradiation to the treatment of malignant disease. The biological effects characteristic of exposure to irradiation were recognized soon after the discovery of X-rays in 1895. The effect of ionizing irradiation is to deliver energy, measured in photons, to the tissues under treatment.

EFFECTS OF IRRADIATION

The therapeutic effects of irradiation are not due to cauterization or the temperature reached in the tissues. When photons of sufficiently high energy interact with tissues electrons are produced by three processes the predominant interaction depending on the energy of the incident photon beam and on the atomic number of the absorbing material. The ionization produced by these electrons damages the cells by impairing their ability to reproduce.

Considered from the point of view of the physicochemical effects of irradiation, when ionizing irradiation interacts with a target it may do so by a 'direct' or 'indirect' action. 'Direct' action describes the primary ionization of important macromolecules in the biological target and 'indirect' action describes the effect of reactive species produced in water in the biological system which secondarily ionize the sensitive biological targets. The breakdown of water produces five highly reactive products of which the two most important are the hydroxyl radical, which is an oxidizing agent, and the aqueous electron which is a free electron surrounded by a capsule of water molecules which is a powerful reducing agent. These products react with biological targets in the cell, leading to disruption and possibly irreversible damage to the macromolecule.

275

Initially, radiotherapy used X-rays which produced low photon energy, but as a result of developments brought about in part by World War II, such machines have now been displaced. Present-day machines make use of gamma rays from radioactive cobalt 60 sources, and high energy photon and electron beams from linear accelerators.

Until 1954, the unit of absorbed dose was known as a 'rad', being equal to the absorption of 100 erg/g of tissue. In the newer SI terms, the standard adopted is now the Gray (Gy), which is equivalent to 1 joule/kg or 100 rads.

The advantages of the newer, high-energy machines are:

1. A high dose of radiation can be delivered deep within the tissues.
2. High energy irradiation has a skin-sparing effect, the maximum dose of irradiation being several centimetres below the surface thus sparing the particularly sensitive epidermal layers of the skin. Prior to World War II, these layers would be so badly damaged as a result of the low energy irradiation used that they themselves, in the course of time, might undergo malignant change.
3. There is less differential absorption between different tissues.

At a biochemical level the result of irradiation is to ionize strong chemical bonds resulting in the almost instantaneous formation of highly reactive chemical species. These, formed at specific sites within the cells, lead through biochemical intracellular pathways to detectable radiation damage which may take hours or days to express itself and perhaps only after several generations of cell division.

Cellular damage may be expressed by:

1. Failure of the irradiated cell or its progeny to complete mitosis.
2. Early tissue damage due to inability of the irradiated cells to maintain by cell division a number of functional cells, eg. leucopenia following whole body irradiation.
3. Late tissue damage consisting of fibrosis, as occurs in the lung, resulting from either early cell or tissue damage, or later, non-specific changes in the vasculature and non-dividing parenchymal cells, as for example a stricture of the bowel.
4. Genetic damage leading to:
   a. possible malignant transformation.
   b. teratogenic effects.

   c. reproductive cells leading to mutagenic effects on the
offspring.

Dose/response relationship

The exact relationship between the dose given and the fraction of
cells sterilized in a tumour or the fraction of cells which retain their
reproductive integrity in a normally renewable tissue is fundamental to the radiobiological basis of radiotherapy.

    The dose/response curve for mammalian cells has a character-
istic slope. With a small dose, an initial shoulder denoting the
progressive accumulation of sublethal injury occurs, this area being
known as the quasi threshold Dq̇. With a larger dose, the resistance to sterilization is largely overcome and the survival curve
becomes exponential, i.e. a straight line when the fraction of cells
surviving irradiation is plotted on a logarithmic scale against dose
on a linear scale, equal increments of dose producing similar levels
of depopulation. The steepness of this exponential slope is
measured by 1/Dô where Dô is known as the mean lethal dose.
Biological research has shown that there is only a small range of
Dô values for mammalian cells ranging from 100–400 cGy, and in
culture ranging from 150–200 cGy. Another finding of clinical
relevance is that the mean lethal dose 9Dô of normal and tumour
cells, from the same tissue of origin, are similar.

    There is no consistent difference in the radiosensitivity of
normal and tumour cells. Differences in radiosensitivity cannot,
therefore, explain the ability of radiotherapy to eradicate tumours
whilst the surrounding tissues are preserved.

FACTORS AFFECTING CELL RESPONSE

Phase of cell cycle

One important biological point determining the sensitivity of cells
to the effects of irradiation is their phase in the cell cycle. Cells in
mitosis are most susceptible to irradiation, whilst cells in the S
phase, at which time DNA synthesis is occurring, are most resistant. The mean lethal dose (Dô) for malignant cells in mitosis is
about three times lower than that for cells in the S phase.
Unfortunately, whilst it is obvious that radiotherapy should be
synchronized with the life cycle of the cell, this has not proved
possible. Indeed, a further factor enters the equation in that large

numbers of cells capable of division pass into the resting phase, known as the Go phase, in which there is an even greater resistance to irradiation. Thus even in the bone marrow, which may be regarded as a highly active cellular system, it is estimated that 20–50% of the whole population is in the Go phase at any one time.

Fractionation

Because the difference in sensitivity to irradiation of malignant and normal cells is so small, single large doses of irradiation designed to ablate a tumour in one treatment would cause damage to both types of tissue, and so it is standard practice to give the prescribed dose in a series of fractions. By fractionation, the radiotherapist attempts to increase the selective depopulation of the tumour whilst minimizing the cell loss in normal tissues. The raison d'etre for this technique is that the majority of tumour cells have a much longer doubling time than do normal cells. An interval between doses of radiotherapy therefore allows some differential repopulation of the normal tissues that have been included in the treatment volume. By this means the radiotherapist hopes to achieve a better therapeutic ratio, i.e. a maximum cytotoxic effect on the tumour with a minimum morbidity within normal tissues.

Oxygenation

One feature which immediately affects the survival of cells following irradiation is the degree of oxygenation. Most normal cells are 2–3 times more sensitive to irradiation than are hypoxic cells. Even the smallest of clinically detectable tumours probably contains over 10% or more of hypoxic cells, markedly reducing the effectiveness of a single dose of irradiation. However, using small fractionated doses, the initial sterilization of the more sensitive, well-oxygenated cells probably provokes the reoxygenation of surviving hypoxic cells, which will then tend to respond more favourably during the later stages of treatment. However, the exact mechanism of the 'oxygen effect' remains to be elucidated.

Dosage

The physical dose used varies from 20–90 Gy, the majority of tumours given between 40 and 60 Gy. Treatment is being normally given 5 days a week, and the majority of dose prescriptions comply with the Ellis dose relationship:

$$TD = NSD \times N^{0.24} \times T^{0.4}$$

where TD is the prescribed dose, N is the number of fractions, T is the overall treatment time and NSD is the normal standard dose.

Radiobiologically, the normal standard dose is equivalent to a single dose above which the accepted limit of tissue tolerance is exceeded. Besides the direct, or more often implicit, use of NSD, radiotherapy doses are also modified according to the volume requiring treatment.

TUMOUR RESPONSE

In some tumours, particularly those of the haemopoetic system, cell death is almost immediate and the tumour resolves rapidly. In highly differentiated tumours, such as squamous carcinoma, on the other hand, resolution may take several weeks, the difference in clinical response being largely determined by the growth fraction of the tumour. However, the speed of response is in no way indicative of radiocurability, which is frequently determined by the limitations set by the contiguous normal tissues or by the fact that the tumour may well have metatasized prior to adequate treatment of the primary tumour, as is the case with many malignant tumours of the breast.

NORMAL TISSUE RESPONSE

The time and degree of radiation response within normal tissues varies widely, and the dose tolerated by normal tissue depends primarily on the proliferative nature of the component cell population. Thus, normal tissues are more responsive to irradiation if they have a high rate of cellular turnover, a large potential for cell division, as in embryonic tissues, and a low degree of morphological or functional differentiation, as in the testes.

Whole body irradiation in man is usually followed by death within 48 hours if a dose of 100–1000 Gy is received; if the dose is between 10 and 100 Gy, vomiting and diarrhoea occur immediately, subsiding in 2–3 days but followed by a repetition accompanied by dehydration and death within three to five days. A dose of 3–10 Gy in the absence of medical intervention usually causes death within 30 days. A progressive lymphopenia accompanied by diminished ability to produce antibodies increases the chances of infection, and thrombocytopenia leads to petechiae and bleeding.

In those individuals who survive whole body irradiation or children accidently irradiated in utero, there is an increased risk of leukaemia, a risk which appears to diminish after 10 years. In patients in whom radiation dermatitis has occurred, 10–25% will develop skin cancers at a later date, often after many years.

METHODS OF DELIVERY

Apart from conventional beam therapy, radioactive materials may be: implanted within cavities, as in the treatment of gynaecological malignancy, implanted into the tissues and surrounding tissues, interstitial treatment, or given orally or intravenously as in the treatment of thyrotoxicosis or polycythaemia rubra vera.

Examples of materials used for interstitial irradiation are, Gold 198 (half-life 2.7 days), Irridium 192 (half-life 74 days), Radium 226 (half-life 1600 years), Yttrium 90 (half-life 64 hours). These various materials may be incorporated into wires, pins, needles or rods or used as colloidal suspensions. Those materials with a long half-life must be removed, whereas those with a short half-life can be left in situ. Reactive implants were in very common use until after World War II, when the introduction of high-energy cobalt units and linear accelerators so improved external irradiation that the method was almost abandoned. However in some centres, particularly in the United States, they still play a prominent role in therapy.

USE OF RADIOTHERAPY

Tumours primarily treated by irradiation rather than surgery

At the present time, irradiation is used as the primary form of treatment in a number of tumours. These include malignancies of the:

1. Skin.
2. Lips, oropharynx and larynx.
3. Bladder, if adequate removal cannot be achieved by transurethral resection.
4. Brain.
5. Localized lymphomata, e.g. Hodgkin's disease.

6. Cervix, unless local conditions such as a narrow vagina or associated surgical condition make optimal radiotherapy difficult.

Preoperative radiotherapy

Numerous trials are currently in progress to establish the value of preoperative irradiation, particularly in relation to carcinoma of the rectum and breast. At the present time, osteogenic sarcoma are normally treated by radiotherapy prior to advocating radical surgery to the limb.

Postoperative radiotherapy

Postoperative radiotherapy has been shown to alter significantly the prognosis in certain tumours. These include:

1. Germ cell tumours of the testis, in which radiotherapy is given to the regional and juxtaregional lymph nodes after orchidectomy. The field includes the homolateral inguinal, pelvic and para-aortic nodes up to the xiphisternum.
2. Breast tumours, when axillary node biopsy has revealed their involvement.
3. Wilm's tumours of the kidney in childhood, when excision reveals that local spread has occurred.

Palliative radiotherapy

Palliative radiotherapy can be used:

1. To relieve pain. This is particularly successful in the treatment of bone metastases arising from primary tumours of the breast, prostate and lungs.
2. To produce temporary healing of ulcerating tumours associated with malodourous discharge. Relief can be obtained by this means in tumours of the breast, lower rectum and anus.
3. To relieve compression in patients suffering from superior caval compression due to extensive bronchial carcinoma.

25 Ultrasonography and surgical diagnosis

Ultrasound was first applied to the problems of surgical diagnosis in the early 1950s and since then has made rapid strides. It was used extensively firstly in obstetrical practice and then across the whole field of surgical endeavour, so that the examples of its diagnostic capability described in this chapter represent only a fraction of its potential. Little has escaped exploration by this new tool, except for the pulmonary and skeletal systems which, for technical reasons, cannot be investigated by this technique.

BASIC PRINCIPLES

Ultrasound is energy in the form of mechanical vibrations at a frequency higher than those to which the human ear is sensitive, i.e. greater than 20 000 Hz (20 kHz; 1 Hz = 1 cycle of sound per second). The operating range of most diagnostic ultrasonic frequencies lies between 2.5 and 7.5 MHz (1 MHz = 1 000 000 Hz).

Generation of ultrasound

Ultrasound used for diagnostic purposes is generated and detected by the peizoelectric effect, a process involving the converson of electrical to mechanical energy. This effect was discovered by J. and P. Currie in 1880, who observed that the compression of certain crystalline materials produced an electric discharge when the crystal had been cut in planes parallel to those natural to the crystal. Piezoelectric materials are called transducers because they provide a coupling between electrical and mechanical energy. The electric charges bound within the ionic lattice of the material are arranged in such a way that they can react with an applied electric field to produce a mechanical effect, and vice-versa.

Many naturally occurring crystals are piezoelectric, e.g. quartz and lithium sulphate, but the most commonly used material for ultrasonic diagnostic probes is the synthetic ceramic lead zurconate titanate PTZ, which belongs to a group of materials known as the ferroelectrics. To create the piezoelectric characteristic of PTZ, following its initial formation at very high temperatures it is reheated to a temperature of 193 °C (its Curie point); it is then cooled with the application of a high DC voltage, which aligns the anisotropic molecules in the direction of the polarizing electric field. Once polarized in this manner, the ceramic cannot be reheated to the Curie point or it will be depolarized and the piezo-electric characteristics lost. Stimulated by an electric driving force, this element sends waves in both directions; the unwanted wave passing in the opposite direction to the patient must be absorbed in the backing or it will produce interference.

The coupling medium between the patient and the transducer is an important part of the system. In practice, one of the commonest causes of poor results is the use of insufficient coupling material. An adequate amount of this material eliminates any air gap or air bubbles which have a reflection coefficient approaching 100%, thus decreasing the transmitted sound waves to practically zero. Either mineral oil or water soluble gels can be used, the latter lasting longer but being more expensive.

Application of ultrasound

Ultrasonic energy travels in the form of waves causing the particles of the media through which it passes to oscillate about their average positions. As the sound energy passes through the various tissues of the body, it interacts by reflection, refraction, defraction, scattering and adsorption, the type of interaction depending upon the characteristics of the material, the frequency of the wave, the wavelength relative to the size of the object, the orientation of the acoustic interfaces and the acoustic impedance. The result of these various factors produces attenuation of the sound wave; in general, the longer the path over which the sound wave travels, the greater is the attenuation.

When the ultrasonic wave strikes an interface between two media, particularly in a perpendicular axis, the incident sound may be reflected or transmitted. Striking the interface with an oblique incidence, the sound wave will be refracted or, if the wave strikes a heterogenous medium, the wave will be scattered. It is basically the reflected wave which produces the diagnostic capability of ultrasonography. Low-frequency waves have a greater penetrating power than do high frequency waves but produce less definition.

There are various ways in which the information derived from the behaviour of the sound wave can be displayed. The primary display mode, introduced in 1972, was the brightness mode (B-mode) display which gives a two-dimensional cross-sectional representation of the tissues examined on horizontal and vertical axes, while encoding the echo amplitude information in gray levels of between 1 and 14. In this type of imaging, the ultrasound probe is moved across the surface of the body and is a type of scanning particularly suitable for the examination of the abdomen and its contents.

The newer and now almost universally accepted method is real-time ultrasonography. This is performed by means of a self-sweeping probe which produces about 40 B-scan images per second so that the examiner perceives a continuum of motion. Thus, whereas using the older method the aorta appeared in static representation, the examiner is now able to see the systolic dilatation and diastolic diminution in diameter.

The transducers are small and hand-held and thus easily and quickly guided over the skin and angled in various ways so that an entire organ can be examined quickly and efficiently, e.g. a complete examination of the urinary tract may take no more than 10 minutes.

DIAGNOSTIC CAPABILITY

Apart from the lungs (which contain air) and bone, virtually every tissue in the body can be investigated by ultrasonography. In some areas, e.g. the gall bladder and renal tract, ultrasonography is now the first line of investigation. The conditions described below are therefore merely examples of the diagnostic capability of this technique.

Hepato-biliary system

Liver

The liver is scanned through the 'acoustic window' which lies between the lung above and the air-containing colon inferiorly.

The patient inspires deeply and the transducer is angled under the right costal margin. The scans are made in a series of parasagittal planes. A section taken 20 mm to the left of the midline shows the aorta posteriorly and the left lobe of the liver anteriorly; 20 mm to the right of the midline the lumen of the inferior vena cava can be seen, with the portal vein lying somewhat anteriorly as it ascends towards the hilum of the liver. The sensitivity of the method is such that the increased diameter of the portal vein, which occurs in cirrhosis, can easily be recognized.

The common discrete abnormalities of the liver detectable by ultrasonography include metastatic disease, abscess formation, cystic disease and primary hepatoma.

a. Hepatic metastases. Metastatic lesions of the liver can present with a variety of ultrasonic patterns, e.g. there can be a decrease in the echo amplitude compared to that of the rest of the liver, or a metastasis can be highly echogenic. The majority of hepatic tumours, whether primary or secondary, do not have a characteristic echo pattern, although metastases arising from primary colonic tumours tend to be hyperechoic, possibly due to their vascularity and mucinous nature. Lymphomata of the liver tend to produce such low echo levels that they simulate intrahepatic abscesses.

b. Abscesses within the liver or in the right suprahepatic space produce relatively sonolucent areas, the amplitude of the echo depending upon the fluidity of the abscess contents. If the abscess is in the upper part of the right lobe or right suprahepatic space, the presence of fluid within the pleural cavity can also be shown. The ability to localize abscesses in this way means that with the aid of ultrasonography abscesses can be drained without open operation, drainage being accomplished by an indwelling plastic tube or by intermittent aspiration.

c. Cysts. Cysts of the liver may be either congenital or acquired. The former appear as well-defined structures with smooth walls, and from within the cyst there is a total absence of echoes due to the non-reflective nature of the fluid within the cyst. In contrast, echinococcal cysts produce varying findings depending upon the different stages of development.

d. Primary liver tumours. Primary hepatomata produce homogenous irregular areas with poorly defined borders and occasional internal echoes which, if present, indicate necrotic degeneration.

e. Generalized hepatic disease. Cirrhosis can be reliably

diagnosed by ultrasonography, because the cirrhotic liver in which fibrosis has occurred returns higher echo levels than does the normal hepatic tissue. Penetration is, however extremely poor, due to severe attentuation caused by the fibrosis.

Biliary tract

a. A distended gall bladder. This, of course, may be caused by the development of a mucocoele due to a calculus blocking the cystic duct, in which case the calculus will be clearly seen. It may, however, be due to a lesion involving the common duct, in which case the common duct itself will be seen to be dilated beyond the normally accepted diameter of 6 mm. If the investigator is then able to trace the duct distally, the site and the cause of the obstruction may be identified. Traced proximally, the dilated intrahepatic ducts can normally be seen. The diagnosis of extrahepatic jaundice due to biliary obstruction can be confirmed in nearly every patient, the distinction between extra- and intrahepatic obstruction being made solely on the differing dimensions of the hepatic and common bile ducts.

b. Gallstones can be visualized even when they are radiolucent. A marked shadowing effect may be seen beyond a stone due to severe attentuation of the beam during its passage through the stone or stones.

The advantages of ultrasonography in hepato-biliary disease are:

1. It is a rapidly performed non-invasive technique.
2. Conventional oral or intravenous cholangiograms are unlikely to be successful in the presence of clinical jaundice.
3. Both percutaneous cholangiography, even when performed with a Chiba needle, and/or endoscopic retrograde cholangiography are not without risk, and both are certainly more costly and time consuming.

The pancreas

Examination of the distal part of the body and tail of the pancreas is difficult because they lie behind the stomach and transverse colon, but the head and most of the body can be visualized by making use of the acoustic window. Normal pancreatic tissue produces an area of homogenous stippled appearance, the echo amplitude being somewhat higher that those of normal liver. The normal pancreatic duct can also be seen and, in a healthy gland, should be no more than 3 mm in diameter.

   a. Pancreatic tumours. Tumours of this organ must be some 3–4 cm in diameter before they can be distinguished from the normal surrounding tissue, when they will appear as irregular masses.

   b. Pancreatitis. Both acute and chronic pancreatitis can be recognized on ultrasonography because the development of oedema increases the permeability of the organ to sound, its outlines becoming easier to detect. The inflamed pancreas presents with an outline greater than that of the normal gland, the body of which normally measures 2.5 ± 0.3 cm with very low level echoes.

   A relatively common complication of pancreatitis is the development of pseudocysts, which can be easily recognized as echo-free masses lying adjacent to the body or tail of the pancreas. If this diagnosis is suspected the stomach should be completely empty before commencing the examination, otherwise confusion may arise because a dilated fluid filled stomach can produce a similar picture.

Urogenital tract

The kidneys, lying in the retroperitoneal tissues, are 'covered' anteriorly by gas-filled loops of bowel. In consequence, direct 'vision' through the peritoneal cavity is diffcult. However, by using the acoustic window provided by the liver, both the right and left kidneys may be scanned.

   A longitudinal scan of a normal kidney shows the readily recognizable oval, smooth outline of the kidney, with the calices, pelvis and blood vessels forming a central group of high amplitude echoes. When the scan passes lateral to the calices, no central echo can be found. In transverse scans, the normal kidney is obviously oval or rounded in shape, and the calices produce a group of echoes which are nearly central in position when the scan passes through one of the renal poles, or is medially placed if the scan goes through the renal pelvis. Above and below the calices, the central echo is absent and the ureters are unidentifiable unless they are dilated.

   a. Renal cell carcinoma. A renal tumour normally indents, displaces or destroys a part of the kidney and caliceal system, so that the organ loses its regular outline. It is replaced by a mass which, because of its heterogenicity, produces multiple random echoes, the necrotic parts of the neoplasm having a very low echogenicity in comparison with the solid areas. These findings are quite distinct to those found when a renal cyst is present. A cyst is usually well defined and, in addition, because of the homogenous nature of its contents, no echoes arise from within the cyst because the ultrasonic wave is only slightly attenuated.

b. Hydronephrosis. The diagnosis of hydronephrosis by ultrasonography depends on the degree of pelvic dilatation which, in turn, produces separation of the central echoes. This causes a ring of echoes in a longitudinal scan, and in advanced cases, particularly those in which there is a large element of extrarenal hydronephrosis, the dilated pelvis can be identified as a transonic mass lying medial to the kidney. Should the cause be an impacted stone at any point in the ureter, this will cause an area of dense echogenicity in an otherwise anechoic area, and distal to the stone will be the usual ultrasonic shadowing.

Ultrasonography can also be used to establish the presence and volume of the residual urine in a patient suffering from prostatism or an atonic bladder. By the use of intrarectal probes the size of the prostate and the presence of extraprostatic spread, if the prostate is malignant, can be identified.

c. Bladder tumours. The presence or absence of infiltration of the bladder wall in patients suffering from malignant tumours of the bladder can also be determined by ultrasonography. In performing this examination the bladder should be full.

Brain

The range of structures that lie in the median sagittal plane from the surface of the scalp can be measured by means of midline echoencephalopathy. A significant difference in the ranges measured from either side of the head suggests that the cerebral midline structures have been displaced, although it may not be possible to determine the precise nature of the lesion responsible for such a displacement. A midline shift following an acute injury is most commonly caused by an intracranial haemorrhage or subdural haematoma.

In a patient suffering from a head injury causing severe generalized cerebral oedema, the interhemispheric fissure tends to be obliterated as the interfaces on either side of it are pressed together. The result is that the echogenicity of this interface is reduced and may not be easily identified. It is for this reason that, when performing midline echoencephalography, the investigator must be aware of the full clinical history and the potential under-lying pathology.

In chronic conditions, the displacement may be the result of a brain tumour or, alternatively, the midline may be drawn to the affected side by an atrophic lesion such as an old clot or cerebral infarct.

So far as the brain is concerned, ultrasonography has now been replaced, in those hospitals in which the apparatus is available, by computer assisted axial tomography which, like ultrasonography, is a non-invasive technique.

Cardiovascular system

The cardiovascular system can be examined by making use of the Doppler effect. When a beam of ultrasound is reflected from a stationary surface, the returning beam is of the same frequency as the generated beam. However, if the reflecting surface is moving, the returning beam has a different frequency from the generated beam – the 'Doppler shift' – and the change in frequency is propor-tional to the velocity of the moving structure.

Using this principle, the activity of the myocardium and its state, the function of the aortic and mitral valves and the presence or absence of functional derangements can be discerned. As a result, echocardiography has largely displaced invasive means of measuring the pressure differentials on either side of these struc-tures.

Similarly, the degree of dilalation or stenosis and the presence or absence of atheroma can be ascertained in the aorta and peripheral vessels.

COMPUTERIZED AXIAL TOMOGRAPHY AND NUCLEAR MAGNETIC RESONANCE

The impact of ultrasonography in surgical practice cannot be overstated. However, even greater potential to visualize patholog-ical change in the intact human has come with the development, beginning in the early 1970s, of two different imaging devices: computerized axial tomography (CAT) by Hounsfield, and at about the same time, nuclear magnetic resonance (NMR; also known as magnetic resonance imaging, (MRI) by Damadian.

One of the major limitations of the normal X-ray is that the shadows cast by a three-dimensional object have to be superimposed on a two-dimensional image plane. Tomography improves the diagnostic capability of the conventional X-ray by recording information from a prescribed slice of the patient on an X-ray plate. Following this advance, computerized axial tomography was developed which, using computers to manipulate the signals produced by photons, allows transverse slices of the body to be produced no more than a few mm in width.

Nuclear magnetic resonance (NMR) works on an entirely different principle. The physical basis is the nuclear magnetization produced by spinning nuclei that contain an odd number of protons, such as hydrogen, lithium, carbon, fluorine and phosporus. When placed in a magnetic field, these nuclear magnets try to realign themselves within it. If a radiofrequency pulse of energy is now applied, the tiny magnetic nuclear fields are destabilized but, following this, once more realign themselves. In so doing, they emit their own radiofrequency signal and it is this signal which is recorded and then processed by computer to produce a visible image of the tissues under examination.

Whereas with CAT the majority of work must be performed in transverse section, with NMR the slice orientation can be in any plane.

26 Diagnostic and therapeutic uses of radionuclides

Isotopes are variants of an element that contain the same number of protons but a different number of neutrons within the nucleus. Difference in the number of neutrons produces an element that is indistinguishable chemically but one which has a nucleus that is unstable and, therefore, liable to undergo spontaneous disintegration, resulting in the release of alpha, beta, or gamma particles.

Detection of emission

Alpha, beta or gamma particles can be detected by a variety of different methods, e.g. photographic film, ionization detectors, geiger counters, or scintillation detectors. Scintillation detectors, which are in common use, convert irradiation into photons of visible or ultraviolet light by interaction with crystals such as sodium iodide.

SURGICAL APPLICATIONS OF ISOTOPES

Isotope studies have been applied to the solution of surgical problems in four ways:

1. For tumour detection.
2. For the visual recording of the progress of a disease.
3. As a test of organ function.
4. As therapeutic agents.

Bone scans

Bone scans are most frequently used to detect metastases in bone which are not visible on simple radiographic examination, particularly in patients suffering from carcinoma of the breast or prostate.

The majority of agents used for bone scanning involve interchange with the bone mineral, hydroxyapatite, rather than the organic matrix. The aim of a bone scan is to provide a picture of radionuclide accumulation in new crystal formation, new crystals forming whenever there is a lesion in bone, whether benign, malignant or inflammatory, because the reaction of bone tissue is to form new bone at the periphery of the lesion or at its actual site.

For several years an analogue of calcium, strontium 85 (^{85}Sr) was used, more recently ^{99m}Tc-labelled phosphorus-containing compounds have been introduced, of which ^{99m}Tc-diphosphonate is an agent in wide use. The mechanism of uptake is not yet fully clear but it may be associated with replacement of the hydroxyapatite crystal of calcium and/or hydroxyl ions.

The uptake of a bone-seeking nuclide is governed by three major factors:

1. The rate of substitution of the isotope used for stable calcium and hydroxyl ions; this reaction probably occurs in amorphous calcium phosphate which is a precursor of hydroxapatite.
2. Bone blood flow, which influences the delivery of an isotope into areas of activity.
3. Hormonal influences, because these govern the quantitative aspects of mineralization.

^{85}Sr can be detected on a bone scan when its local concentration has reached approximately three times the normal value. Any reactive process within the bone that results in either a translucency or increased density on the plain radiograph always produces an abnormal scan.

One of the chief advantages of isotope scanning is that abnormalities in the calcium content of a bone can be detected by this means much sooner than by a plain X-ray, often by several months, because changes in the latter occur only after the calcium content has fallen by 30–50%.

However, the changes observed on a bone scan are wholly non-specific. Other conditions producing positive scans include benign tumours, arthritides, Paget's disease, dysplasia, fractures, synovitis, soft tissue inflammation and osteoporosis. A skeletal fracture is followed by an increased uptake of isotope for two to three years.

Thus an examination should always be preceded by a careful history, physical examination, and the performance of those biochemical tests which normally indicate bone disease, if abnormal. These tests include measurement of the serum calcium and urinary calcium excretion, the alkaline phosphatase, and the urinary creatinine/hydroxyproline ratio.

Isotopic surveys of the skeleton may be used by the surgeon in one of two ways: for screening apparently well women, or for the confirmation of already suspected bone lesions.

Isotope scanning of the skeleton for women suffering from breast cancer

This became popular in the early 1970s, when different investigators reported that in clinically early cases as many as 45% of women might have a positive scan. However, there was a wide variation between different hospitals; the British Breast Group, for example, reporting the results from eight centres, found that the range of positive bone scans in surgically treatable disease varied between 2 and 20% with an average of 10%, this in patients who had no skeletal symptoms.

In a series in which the patient was later followed up, it was found that only about 50% developed osseous metastases, a fact which emphasizes that therapeutic decisions should not be based on bone scan findings alone. Thus, the false-positive rate is as high as 50%.

Whilst opinions vary, there is little evidence to support the performance of routine bone scans prior to surgery. The clinico-pathological features which imply that patients may develop osseous metastases are as follows:

1. Positive nodes at the time of operation.
2. The higher in the axilla the involved nodes, the greater is the chance of developing osseous metastases.
3. The larger the diameter of the primary lesion the greater the chance of osseous metastases.
4. Younger patient. Osseous metastases develop twice as commonly in premenopausal as compared to postmenopausal females.

Negative bone scan

A scan may sometimes be negative even in the presence of a bony lesion if there is rapid bone destruction without any associated reactive osteogenesis. Conversely, stable secondaries, which sometimes occur in thyroid cancer, may also produce little if any observable changes.

Brain scans

Brain scanning can now be effectively used for:

1. The diagnosis of intracranial space-occupying lesions.
2. The estimation of cerebral blood flow.

The following isotopes have been used: ^{99m}Tc, ^{197}Hg-chlormerodin and ^{113m} indium chelate. Iodinated macroaggregated albumin has also been used, but this is potentially dangerous because of the particle size which is such that it may block the cerebral arterioles.

Tumour diagnosis

Three factors largely determine whether a tumour can be identified by scanning techniques:

1. The differential uptake pattern.
2. The location of the tumour.
3. The size of the tumour.

Peripheral tumours lying within normal brain tissue are more easily distinguished from normal brain tissue than are central tumours such as pinealomas, and the vascular pattern at the base of the skull frequently makes tumours in this area difficult to locate. In terms of pathology, meningiomas, glioblastomas and metastatic lesions are more easily located than the less vascular astrocytomas.

Estimation of cerebral blood flow

This investigation is of particular interest to the surgeon when considering the clinical significance of carotid artery stenosis.

Liver scans

The commonest use of a liver scan is to detect the presence of metastases from primary tumours elsewhere in the body. The most commonly used isotope is ^{99m}Tc. This technique will identify defects in the liver over 2 cm in diameter, but a scan alone will not differentiate between an abscess, cyst or neoplastic lesion. Some help may be obtained by additional use of ultrasonography which will identify lesions of similar size but with slight differences in echogenicity which may be more informative.

Nevertheless, even using both techniques with small lesions in the liver, a high percentage of false-negatives has been reported by different observers and, conversely, a relatively high percentage of false-positive results occurs. Thus, many investigators would suggest that a liver scan should be used to create an index of suspicion. However, if secondary metastases from colorectal cancer are suspected (Fig. 26.1) the accuracy of a scan is markedly improved if the carcinoembryonic antigen level is also elevated.

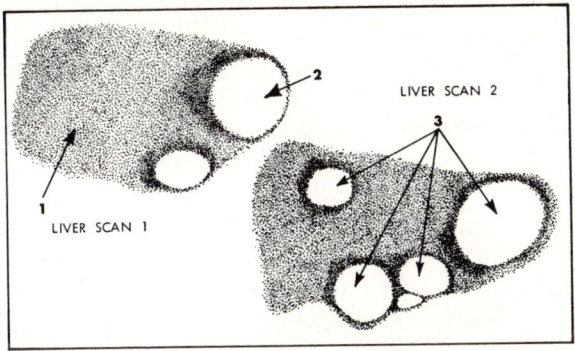

Fig. 26.1   Serial liver scan showing progressive development of defects from secondary deposits arising from a carcinoma of the colon.
1. Liver substance
2. Defect
3. Multiple defects seen several months later.

A liver scan combined with a lung scan is of considerable value in detecting a right suprahepatic abscess when no air is present in the abscess cavity. Such a technique demonstrates a silent area between the parenchyma of the lung and the liver which represents the space occupied by the abscess. Drainage leading to cure of the abscess leads to approximation of the two scans.

Lung scans

A large number of different types of pulmonary and pleural masses can be demonstrated by isotope scanning of the lungs but, as in other areas, a scan, whilst demonstrating the defect in the lung fields, gives little or no indication of the precise diagnosis.

In the surgical patient, a common indication for the use of isotopic techniques is in the diagnosis of pulmonary embolus. If this condition is suspected and a perfusion scan alone performed, a number of false-positive results will occur due to the presence of primary pulmonary disease. However, the majority of these conditions are associated with an abnormal chest X-ray, whereas the radiography even in the presence of a massive pulmonary embolus merely shows pulmonary oligaemia. Therefore, to reduce, the number of false-positive diagnoses, the perfusion scan should be followed by a ventilation scan.

The common agent used for perfusion scanning is labelled macroaggregated albumin, the isotope label being provided by ^{99m}Tc, ^{133}In or ^{51}Cr. The macroaggregated albumin is large enough to lodge in the pulmonary capillaries following intravenous injection, with the result that the subsequent scan reflects the pattern of perfusion.

The posture of the patient is important because the pulmonary circulation is a low-pressure system. In the erect position, the lung fields are increasingly dense from the apices to the bases. To achieve an even distribution of the isotope through the pulmonary circulation, it should be injected slowly with the patient in either the supine or erect position. Four standard projections are normally taken: the posterior, anterior, and right and left lateral. The posterior view is regarded as the most important because it encompasses the greatest volume of lung; in lateral views the opposite lung makes a 30% contribution to the image.

The characteristic abnormality indicating the presence of a pulmonary embolus is a segmental defect caused by the perfusion defect.

The ventilation scan is performed by the inhalation of either krypton-81^m or xenon^{125}, ^{127} or ^{133}. Whilst krypton produces better definition, its half-life of only 13 seconds limits its usefulness. The scan is made after a single deep inspiration. This shows the initial distribution of the inspired air. Alternatively, multiple scans can be made whilst the gas is being continuously breathed in and, later, when it is being expired, so-called wash-in and wash-out scans. A ventilation scan made some hours after an embolus normally shows no defect in the embolized area, even though the perfusion study is grossly abnormal.

Perfusion/ventilation scanning is as sensitive as conventional pulmonary arteriography and being non-invasive, is much safer.

Pancreatic scans

The principles of pancreatic scanning are as follows: firstly, the pancreas may be emptied of its pre-existing enzymes by an injection of secretin and pancreazymin; secondly, the liver is outlined with colloidal ^{198}Au, after which a dose of selenium-tagged methionine is given. ^{75}Se has a half-life of 128 days; it is incorporated into the methionine molecule in place of sulphur, producing a gamma-emitting amino acid. The uptake of selenomethionine is related to the level of enzyme synthesis, and in the first hour after administration about 7% is localized in the pancreas, the maximum uptake being within 30 minutes. In a normal scan, the neck, body and tail assume either a straight or a sigmoid configuration in relation to the head.

This investigation is not often used because there are other, in general terms more effective, investigations. These include retrograde cannulation of the pancreatic duct via the ampulla of Vater in order to perform a retrograde pancreatogram, the use of ultrasound and, lastly, pancreatic arteriography.

Renal scans

The kidney can be investigated by means of radionuclides which are excreted by glomerular filtration and tubular secretion, or by materials bound to the renal cortex.

The former includes suitably labelled water-soluble radiological contrast media or the stable chelates of most metals. The commonly used agents are ^{99m}Tc DTPA (diethylene tetrapentacetic acid) and ortho-iodohippurate labelled with ^{131}I or ^{125}I, 80% of the latter agent being secreted by the renal tubules.

Such materials are almost completely 99% extracted from the blood with each passage through the kidneys and, since 25% of the cardiac output is channelled through the kidneys, within a period of $2\frac{1}{2}$–5 minutes all the above agents rapidly come into view on the gamma camera.

Isotope techniques permit a semiquantitative measurement of the renal blood flow and renal function. In addition, the anatomical size and shape of the kidneys together with information regarding the thickness of the cortical tissue and the size of the pelvis and ureter can be estimated.

The type of clinical problem in which imaging techniques may be helpful are:

1. The determination of unilateral alterations in renal function caused, for example, by renal artery stenosis.
2. The diagnosis of obstructive uropathy and the follow-up of patients treated by operations such as pyeloplasty.
3. The diagnosis of space-occupying lesions.
4. The demonstration of cortical damage by recurrent pyelonephritis.
5. To determine the presence or absence of vesico-ureteric reflux.
6. To assess the function of renal transplants.

Normal renogram (Fig. 26.2)

The normal renogram shows three classical phases, formerly termed the vascular, secretory and excretory slopes but now referred to as the first, second and third phases.

The first phase reflects the rapidity of injection and the vascular supply of the kidney; the radioactivity detected is that in the blood, kidney and extrarenal tissues. The second phase corresponds to the manner in which the isotope is handled by the kidney. Many factors determine the shape of this part of the curve. Essentially, however, the curve rises because more isotope is arriving at the kidney through recirculation but none has left the renal pelvis. Thus, if the patient is suffering from an obstructive uropathy this curve continues to rise. In a normal kidney, however, after $2\frac{1}{2}$–5 minutes the isotope commences to leave the kidney producing a sudden fall in the curve, the third or excretory slope. At about this time tracer activity begins to appear in the bladder.

Diuresis renography is a modification of the standard technique which is particularly valuable in differentiating between significant and harmful obstruction. It can be used to demonstrate the presence of idiopathic hydronephrosis, dilatation of the ureter in primary megaureter or obstruction following reimplantation procedures.

Obstruction of the urinary outflow at the pelviureteric junction causes the normally concave excretory slope (phase 3) to become less concave. When obstruction is complete the original vascular spike (phase 1) continues to rise throughout the duration of the

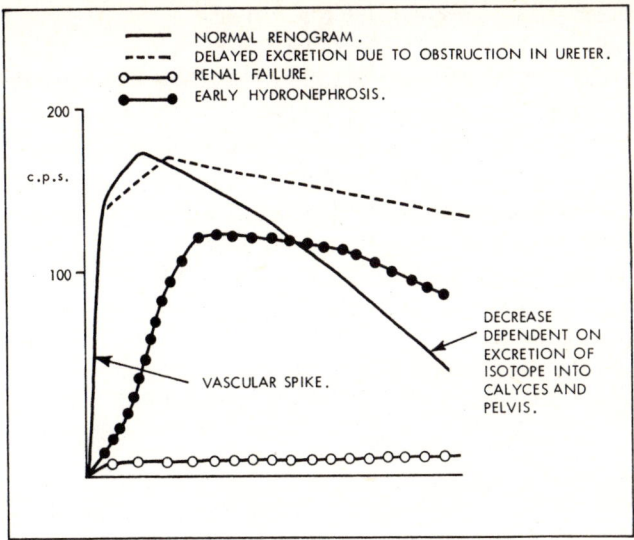

Fig. 26.2 Renogram showing normal and abnormal patterns.

scan until, finally, when the kidney becomes non-functioning, the normal concave slope is converted into a flat or convex configuration.

A distinction between cysts of the kidney and renal neoplasms can also be made by using a gamma camera and visualizing the vascular input into the affected kidney. A rapid intravenous injection of a bolus containing 10 mCi of any 99^m Tc agent is administered, and 50 1-second or 5-second frames are taken beginning 5 seconds after the injection. By this technique the agent can be visualized as it passes through the renal arteries and individual kidneys. A hypervascular blush in this study, corresponding to a defect or 'cold' area in the parenchymal study, is diagnostic of a tumour. This contrasts with a renal cyst in which both parenchymal and vascular studies are 'cold'.

Thyroid scanning and thyroid function

In the recent past, the measurement of the uptake of the various isotopes of iodine by the thyroid was the most commonly used method of estimating thyroid function. These tests have now been almost universally abandoned to be replaced by the direct measurement of the circulating T^4, T^3 and TSH. Furthermore, it has recently been recognized that, in the majority of patients presenting with an apparently solitary nodule of the thyroid, initial ultrasonography is the most useful investigation. By this means, it can be established whether the swelling is cystic or solid. If cystic, there is a possibility that simple aspiration will relieve the condition, although in the author's hands this method has been singularly unsuccessful. Only if the swelling is echo-poor or echo-rich need radionuclide imaging be performed. If this reveals a 'cold' nodule the possibility of malignancy arises, although this danger is not as great as was once thought, 95% at least of cold nodules being benign. If the nodule is 'warm' or 'hot' it may safely be left in situ (or removed if causing thyrotoxicosis).

The common isotopes used in the investigation of the thyroid are ^{99m}Tc, I^{123} and I^{131}.

THERAPEUTIC USE OF ISOTOPES IN CARCINOMA OF THE THYROID

If a thyroid cancer, particularly a metastatic thyroid cancer, can take up ^{131}I, this may form a useful method of treatment. It implies some degree of differentiation of the tumour for the anaplastic carcinomas cannot be treated by this method due to a lack of uptake.

The majority of surgeons would accept that the primary treatment of thyroid cancer is surgical, especially when the cancer is confined to the neck, i.e. involving only the thyroid and the cervical lymph nodes, unless the condition is inoperable as is often the case when the tumour is anaplastic.

A major problem has always been to stimulate extracervical deposits to take up sufficient radioactive isotope for their destruction, and in order to accomplish this all normal thyroid tissue must be destroyed. This can be achieved either surgically by total thyroidectomy, which carries the disadvantage of a high incidence of hypoparathyroidism, or by the use of ^{181}I, 75–150 mCi being administered following an injection of thyroid-stimulating hormone.

Only after the ablation of all normal thyroid tissue does treatment of the metastatic disease begin. However, it is extremely difficult to assess the overall effects of this method of treatment because of the biological variation in the behaviour of thyroid cancer. Both age and the histological appearance of the tumour greatly influence the survival time. McDermott of the

Massachusetts General Hospital found, for example, that regardless of histological type, patients diagnosed and treated prior to the age of 40 did well, with a mortality directly attributable to tumour of 8%, whereas patients over 40 years of age had a mortality of 58%. Similar results have been reported by other workers in this field.

27 Common non-surgical causes of acute abdominal pain

A discussion of the medical causes of abdominal pain might seem inappropriate in a surgical text, but it is essential that a surgeon should be aware of the many medical causes that may mimic a 'surgical abdomen' if unnecessary laparotomy is to be avoided.

COMMON CAUSES IN CHILDHOOD

1. Mesenteric adenitis

This disease is confined to children and is the commonest cause of misdiagnosis in children suspected of suffering from acute appendicitis. Often, the affected child has suffered from a recent upper respiratory tract infection, signs of which may still be present, particularly in the throat. Abdominal pain may begin in the central abdomen but soon becomes localized to the right iliac fossa. The child is always febrile, in contradistinction to early acute appendicitis, and tender in the lower abdomen. When a laparotomy is performed, a mass of enlarged glands are found in the mesentery from which the adenoviruses can be cultured. Later, during convalescence, neutralizing antibodies are found in the serum.

A physical sign said to help in differentiating this condition from appendicitis is the mobility of the point of maximum tenderness. The child is examined supine and the point of maximum tenderness is found by palpation. He is then rolled onto the left side. If the point of tenderness moves medially this is said to favour a diagnosis of mesenteric adenitis rather than appendicitis. This sign should, however, be treated with great caution. The author regards it as useless!

2. Pneumonia

The diagnosis of pneumonia, either bacterial or viral, is often left unconsidered in children, but when it affects the right lower lobe it is a relatively common cause of abdominal pain in childhood. Children under the age of 7 rarely spit and, therefore, the characteristic 'rusty' sputum due to altered blood from areas of red hepatization is not produced. However, in the young child suffering from a pulmonary infection, the pulse/respiration ratio, normally about 4:1, decreases and the alar nasae move in the inspiratory phase of respiration. When the cause of the abdominal pain lies below the diaphragm this ratio usually increases, and the alar nasae move only when general peritonitis is beginning to restrict diaphragmatic movement. These latter observations are of great importance because the abdominal wall may be rigid in both supra- and infradiaphragmatic conditions.

3. Infestation with worms

Many worm infestations remain symptomless or provoke nutritional changes. Those producing attacks of abdominal pain include:

a. The whip worm, *Trichuris trichura*, which inhabits the large intestine and especially the caecum. When there is a severe infection, pain in the right iliac fossa may mimic acute appendicitis.
b. The round worm, *Ascaris lumbricoides*, is especially common in tropical countries, and in some parts of Africa is the commonest cause of abdominal pain in childhood when the worms migrate into either the common bile or pancreatic ducts, producing biliary obstruction or acute pancreatitis.
c. The threadworm, *Enterobius vermicularis*, may well be found within the appendix or even penetrating the wall, but it is extremely doubtful whether it is ever responsible for appendicular pain.

4. The exanthemata

In all the exanthemata the prodromal stage may be associated with acute abdominal distress, e.g. scarlet fever, streptococcal sore throat, mumps and measles.

Intermittent abdominal pain of unknown aetiology also occurs in childhood. This type of pain is seen most frequently between the ages of 8 and 10 and the pain may be so severe that the child is not taken to school or, once there, is brought home. Such pain is often in the periumbilical region and may cause the child to vomit for several hours. When the child localizes the pain to the right iliac fossa, the parents live in constant fear that each attack may herald acute appendicitis. In these circumstances it is often better to remove the appendix, knowing that it will be normal, after carefully explaining to the parents that the attacks of pain may well continue. Occasionally, investigation of such a child leads to the finding of a previously unsuspected duodenal ulcer, Crohn's disease, or a congenital anomaly of the renal tract.

5. Blood disorders

Henoch Schönlein purpura

Classically, this condition is associated with abdominal pain, a skin rash and joint pains. The diagnosis should go unrecognized only if there is no skin rash. This is usually papular at first and purpuric later. The condition affects children usually 7–28 days after an acute respiratory tract infection. The underlying pathological change is in the capillaries which are damaged by an allergic response. As a result, capillary permeability increases and red cells and plasma escape into the surrounding tissues, provoking a perivascular cellular inflammatory reaction. In severe cases a similar lesion in the kidney leads to microscopic haematuria. The abdominal pain is caused by lesions in the bowel. Occasionally, the degree of local irritation is sufficient to induce an intussusception but, more frequently, an ileus develops which leads to repeated vomiting and slowly increasing abdominal distention. Although Henoch's purpura is primarily a medical condition, if an intussusception develops it will require either radiological or surgical reduction.

Sickle cell disease

Sickle cell disease is a common condition in the African negro and descendants from this stock. It is due to the presence of an abnormal haemoglobin in the red cell, known as haemoglobin S. This structural abnormality of the haemoglobin molecule causes it to crystallize into rigid rods when the PaO_2 falls. As a result the red cell twists into the familiar sickle shape.

The effect of this makes the red cells sensitive to trauma and reduces their survival in the circulation and, in addition, the mis-shapen cells tend to migrate to the capillary beds and produce thrombosis. Infarcts occur in the spleen, lungs, and elsewhere and may lead to attacks of abdominal pain, particularly in childhood. The surgeon should be alerted by the skin colour of the patient. A screening test may be positive but this does not necessarily rule out a concomitant surgical emergency.

COMMON CAUSES IN THE ADULT

1. Viral infections

Herpes zoster or shingles

This is a herpetiform eruption affecting sensory nerves and is caused by the same virus as chicken pox. A patient suffering from herpes may transmit chicken pox to a child. Degeneration and demyelination of the posterior horn cells occurs. The first symptom of herpes is usually pain in the cutaneous dermatome of one or more nerve roots. Three to five days later the typical eruption develops. The initial pain of herpes can obviously be mistaken for an acute surgical condition only if the roots between T_7 and L_1 are involved, because these supply the dermatomes with an abdominal distribution. If the T_{10} and T_{11} dermatomes are affected on the right side, the initial pain can easily mimic appendicitis or a twisted ovarian cyst.

Bornholm's disease

This condition, caused by the coxsackie B virus, derives its name from the Danish island on which there was an epidemic. It presents with sudden pain, in the lower chest or upper abdomen, which is severe but intermittent, recurring at intervals, usually for about a week. The area of the abdominal wall in which the pain is felt may be tender and rigid. The disease is usually epidemic and affects, in particular, relatively closed communities such as schools, army barracks, and nurses' homes. It is, therefore, common for the first few patients to go undiagnosed. Similarly, the diagnosis is difficult to reach in an isolated case.

2. Pulmonary causes

As in the child, a right-sided diaphragmatic pleurisy may produce severe right upper abdominal pain, thus mimicking acute cholecystitis or perforated duodenal ulcer.

3. Acute coronary occlusion

This condition is usually associated with severe chest pain, radiating to the neck and arms, which may be severe from the onset or build up in crescendo fashion. Weakness, nausea, and even vomiting can occur. Less frequently, the pain and discomfort begin in the epigastrium and are occasionally accompanied by rigidity, suggesting acute cholecystitis, acute pancreatitis, or a perforated peptic ulcer. These different modes of presentation occur regardless of whether the patient is at rest, excessively active, starving or replete, and only rarely does the patient give a history of increasing angina which would assist in the differential diagnosis.

4. Metabolic disease

Diabetes may cause acute abdominal pain during the initial stages of a diabetic crisis as the patient becomes ketotic. The reason is unknown. The severity of the pain appears to be proportional to the ketosis rather than to the level of the blood sugar. Although ketoacidosis may be the first symptom of diabetes, it is more frequently the result of an acute infection in an established diabetic. The classical signs of ketoacidosis are present and include a dry tongue, rapid weak pulse, and hypotension due to sodium depletion and dehydration. The breath smells of acetone and the urine is loaded with ketone bodies and glucose.

The severity of the condition can be assessed by measuring the plasma bicarbonate concentration, a value of less than 10 mmol/l indicating that the patient is severely acidotic. Because such patients are clinically extremely dehydrated, a total body water deficit of 6 litres being common, there is a certain urgency for administering intravenous fluids. Fortunately for the patients, as the dehydration is corrected so the abdominal pain tends to improve, even in the absence of specific measures such as administration of soluble insulin. This has saved many patients from an unnecessary laparotomy.

5. Blood disorders

Porphyria

Acute intermittent porphyria is an autosomal dominant inherited disease classified into two varieties, the hepatic and erythropoietic. The latter is rare, the first manifestations usually occurring in infancy or childhood. The clinical features associated with hepatic porphyria seldom begin before puberty and consist of episodic attacks of colicky abdominal pain, vomiting, and constipation. Thus, the disease may mimic either small bowel obstruction or acute appendicitis. In keeping with the former diagnosis there may be a number of operation scars. Much less frequently an attack may be associated with lower motor neurone paresis or paralysis, the weakness progressing to a flaccid paraplegia.

The pain of porphyria can be precipitated by many pharmacological agents including oral contraceptives, barbiturates, methyldopa, and alcohol. Since the porphyrins and their precursors are pharmacologically inactive the clinical symptoms are probably due to a neuropathy.

When a patient presents for the first time with this condition, only a high degree of suspicion on the part of the surgeon will lead to the correct diagnosis, unless all patients complaining of acute abdominal pain are routinely screened by the use of Ehrlich's aldehyde reagent (*p*-dimethylaminobenzaldehyde). To 5 ml of this reagent is added 5 ml of urine, after which 10 ml of saturated sodium acetate together with 10 ml of benzylamyl alcohol solution is added. The appearance of an intense red colour indicates the presence of porphyrins. A specimen of urine passed by the patient at the time of admission is normal in colour, and only becomes the classic Burgundy red on standing. This is due to the gradual conversion of colourless prophobilinogen to the red uroporphyrin.

6. Neurological conditions

The gastric crisis of tabes is a cause of abdominal pain. Acute severe intermittent pains are characteristic of tabes dorsalis. Although the pains may affect any part of the body, the surgeon's interest is aroused when the pain is abdominal. At this stage in the disease there is symmetrical degeneration of both axons and myelin of the dorsal columns of the spinal cord. Damage to the somatic sensory fibres leads to paroxysmal pain and to impairment of temperature and pain sensation. Damage to the fibres entering the dorsal columns leads to sensory ataxia, and since the afferent arcs of the tendon reflexes are denervated, there is loss of reflexes and hypotonia. The pains do not, in fact, resemble any recognized type of pain produced by the abdominal viscera themselves as they are too severe, too short in duration, and often described as red hot needles. However, they may be associated with vomiting, tenesmus, and strangury. The bizarre description of the pain should alert the surgeon, as should the presence of Argyll Robertson pupils.

7. Psychological pain

A rare cause of abdominal pain in the adult is Munchausen's syndrome. This condition is most commonly seen in females. The patient complains of pain, often colicky in nature, and the presence of abdominal scars suggests a diagnosis of intestinal obstruction. There is usually no associated increase in peristalsis although the patient mimics abdominal rigidity and makes frequent attempts to vomit. Plain X-rays of the abdomen, if obtained, are negative, and sometimes the patient makes certain they are not obtainable, either by fainting on the way to the department or moving as the film is being exposed.

This condition can only be diagnosed if there is a high level of clinical suspicion, which may only be aroused by the multiplicity of abdominal scars. Usually, these patients admit themselves to different hospitals using a variety of aliases to make their movements difficult to trace.